PN Maternal Newborn Nursing
Review Module Edition 9.0

CONTRIBUTORS

Sheryl Sommer, PhD, RN, CNE
VP Nursing Education & Strategy

Janean Johnson, MSN, RN
Nursing Education Strategist

Sherry L. Roper, PhD, RN
Nursing Education Strategist

Karin Roberts, PhD, MSN, RN, CNE
Nursing Education Coordinator

Mendy G. McMichael, DNP, RN
Nursing Education Specialist and Content Project Coordinator

Judy Drumm DNS, RN, CPN
Nursing Education Specialist

EDITORIAL AND PUBLISHING

Derek Prater
Spring Lenox
Michelle Renner
Mandy Tallmadge
Kelly Von Lunen

CONSULTANTS

Christi Blair, MSN, RN

Intellectual Property Notice

Important Notice to the Reader

User's Guide

Welcome to the Assessment Technologies Institute® PN Maternal Newborn Nursing Review Module Edition 9.0. The mission of ATI's Content Mastery Series® review modules is to provide user-friendly compendiums of nursing knowledge that will:

- Help you locate important information quickly.

- Assist in your learning efforts.

- Provide exercises for applying your nursing knowledge.

- Facilitate your entry into the nursing profession as a newly licensed PN.

Organization

This review module is organized into units covering antepartum, intrapartum, postpartum, and newborn nursing care. Chapters within these units conform to one of three organizing principles for presenting the content:

- Nursing concepts

- Procedures

- Complications of pregnancy

Nursing concepts chapters begin with an overview describing the central concept and its relevance to nursing. Subordinate themes are covered in outline form to demonstrate relationships and present the information in a clear, succinct manner.

Procedures chapters include an overview describing the procedure(s) covered in the chapter. These chapters will provide you with nursing knowledge relevant to each procedure, including indications, interpretations of findings, nursing actions, and complications.

Complications of pregnancy chapters include an overview describing the complication, followed by risk factors. These chapters will cover data collection, including subjective and objective data, and patient-centered care, including nursing care, medications, and health promotion.

Application Exercises

Questions are provided at the end of each chapter so you can practice applying your knowledge. The Application Exercises include NCLEX-style questions, such as multiple-choice and multiple-select items, and questions that ask you to apply your knowledge in other formats, such as by using an ATI Active Learning Template. After the Application Exercises, an answer key is provided, along with rationales for the answers.

NCLEX® Connections

To prepare for the NCLEX-PN, it is important for you to understand how the content in this review module is connected to the NCLEX-PN test plan. You can find information on the detailed test plan at the National Council of State Boards of Nursing's Web site: https://www.ncsbn.org/. When reviewing content in this review module, regularly ask yourself, "How does this content fit into the test plan, and what types of questions related to this content should I expect?"

To help you in this process, we've included NCLEX Connections at the beginning of each unit and with each question in the Application Exercises Answer Keys. The NCLEX Connections at the beginning of each unit will point out areas of the detailed test plan that relate to the content within that unit. The NCLEX Connections attached to the Application Exercises Answer Keys will demonstrate how each exercise fits within the detailed content outline.

These NCLEX Connections will help you understand how the detailed content outline is organized, starting with major client needs categories and subcategories and followed by related content areas and tasks. The major client needs categories are:

- Safe and Effective Care Environment
  - Coordinated Care
  - Safety and Infection Control
- Health Promotion and Maintenance
- Psychosocial Integrity
- Physiological Integrity
  - Basic Care and Comfort
  - Pharmacological Therapies
  - Reduction of Risk Potential
  - Physiological Adaptation

An NCLEX Connection might, for example, alert you that content within a unit is related to:

- Health Promotion and Maintenance
  - Ante/Intra/Postpartum and Newborn Care
    - Evaluate client psychosocial response to pregnancy.

QSEN Competencies

As you use the review modules, you will note the integration of the Quality and Safety Education for Nurses (QSEN) competencies throughout the chapters. These competencies are integral components of the curriculum of many nursing programs in the United States and prepare you to provide safe, high-quality care as a newly licensed PN. Icons appear to draw your attention to the six QSEN competencies:

- Safety: The minimization of risk factors that could cause injury or harm while promoting quality care and maintaining a secure environment for clients, self, and others.
- Patient-Centered Care: The provision of caring and compassionate, culturally sensitive care that addresses clients' physiological, psychological, sociological, spiritual, and cultural needs, preferences, and values.

- Evidence-Based Practice: The use of current knowledge from research and other credible sources, on which to base clinical judgment and client care.

- Informatics: The use of information technology as a communication and information-gathering tool that supports clinical decision-making and scientifically based nursing practice.

- Quality Improvement: Care related and organizational processes that involve the development and implementation of a plan to improve health care services and better meet clients' needs.

- Teamwork and Collaboration: The delivery of client care in partnership with multidisciplinary members of the health care team to achieve continuity of care and positive client outcomes.

Icons

Icons are used throughout the review module to draw your attention to particular areas. Keep an eye out for these icons:

 This icon is used for NCLEX connections.

 This icon is used for content related to safety. When you see this icon, take note of safety concerns or steps that nurses can take to ensure client safety and a safe environment.

 This icon is a QSEN competency that indicates the importance of a holistic approach to providing care.

 This icon, a QSEN competency, points out the integration of research into clinical practice.

 This icon is a QSEN competency and highlights the use of information technology to support nursing practice.

 This icon is used to focus on the QSEN competency of integrating planning processes to meet clients' needs.

This icon highlights the QSEN competency of care delivery using an interprofessional approach.

This icon indicates that a media supplement, such as a graphic, animation, or video, is available. If you have an electronic copy of the review module, this icon will appear alongside clickable links to media supplements. If you have a hardcopy version of the review module, visit www.atitesting.com for details on how to access these features.

Feedback

ATI welcomes feedback regarding this review module. Please provide comments to: comments@atitesting.com.

TABLE OF CONTENTS

UNIT 1   Antepartum Nursing Care

SECTIONS

› Human Reproduction
› Low-Risk, Uncomplicated Pregnancy: Changes During Pregnancy
› Complications of Pregnancy

NCLEX® CONNECTIONS

When reviewing the chapters in this unit, keep in mind the relevant sections of the NCLEX® outline, in particular:

Client Needs: Health Promotion and Maintenance

› Relevant topics/tasks include:
  » Ante/Intra/Postpartum and Newborn Care
    › Provide prenatal care and education.
  » Data Collection Techniques
    › Collect data for health history.
  » Health Promotion/Disease Prevention
    › Teach client about health risks and health promotion.
  » Lifestyle Choices
    › Determine the client's need/desire for contraception.
  » High-Risk Behaviors
    › Provide information to prevent high-risk behaviors or lifestyle choices.

Client Needs: Reduction of Risk Potential

› Relevant topics/tasks include:
  » Diagnostic Tests
    › Reinforce teaching about diagnostic tests.
  » Laboratory Values
    › Monitor the results of maternal and fetal diagnostic tests.
  » Potential for Alterations in Body Systems
    › Identify signs or symptoms of potential prenatal complications.

Client Needs: Basic Care and Comfort

› Relevant topics/tasks include:
  » Nonpharmacological Comfort Interventions
    › Determine the client's need for alternative and/or complementary therapy.
  » Nutrition and Oral Hydration
    › Provide for nutritional needs of clients.
  » Pharmacological Therapies
    › Perform dosage calculations.
    › Identify expected actions/outcomes.

Client Needs: Physiological Adaptation

› Relevant topics/tasks include:
  » Alterations in Body Systems
    › Identify/provide care for complications of prenancy/labor and/or delivery.

chapter 1

Overview

- Contraception refers to strategies or devices used to reduce the risk of fertilization or implantation in an attempt to prevent pregnancy.

- A nurse should determine clients' need/desire for contraception, as well as their preferences. A thorough discussion of benefits, risks, and alternatives of each method should be discussed.

- Sexual partners often make a joint decision regarding a desired preference (vasectomy or tubal ligation). Postpartum discharge instructions should include the discussion of future contraceptive plans.

- Expected outcomes for family planning methods consist of preventing pregnancy until a desired time.

- Nurses should support clients in making the decision that is best for their individual situations.

- Methods of contraception include natural family planning, barrier, hormonal, and intrauterine methods, as well as surgical procedures.

Natural Family Planning Methods

ABSTINENCE	
Definition	› Abstaining from having sexual intercourse eliminates the possibility of sperm entering a woman's vagina.
Client Instructions	› Refrain from sexual intercourse. This method can be associated with saying "no," but it also can incorporate saying "yes" to other gratifying sexual activities, such as affectionate touching, communication, holding hands, kissing, massage, and oral and manual stimulation.
Advantages	› Most effective method of birth control. › Abstinence during fertile periods (rhythm method) can be used, but it requires an understanding of the menstrual cycle and fertility awareness. › Can eliminate the risk of STIs if there is no genitalia contact.
Disadvantages	› Requires self-control
Risks/possible complications/ contraindications	› If complete abstinence is maintained, there are no risks.

COITUS INTERRUPTUS (WITHDRAWAL)

Definition	› Man withdraws penis from vagina prior to ejaculation.
Client Instructions	› Be aware of fluids leaking from the penis prior to ejaculation.
Advantages	› Possible choice for monogamous couples with no other option for birth control, such as those opposed to birth control due to religious conviction.
Disadvantages	› Most ineffective method of contraception. › No protection against STIs.
Risks/possible complications/ contraindications	› Male partner's control can make this an effective method. › Leakage of fluid that contains spermatozoa prior to ejaculation can be deposited in vagina. › Risk of pregnancy.

CALENDAR METHOD

Definition	› A woman records her menstrual cycle by calculating her fertile period based on the assumption that ovulation occurs about 14 days before the onset of her next menstrual cycle, and avoids intercourse during that period. Also taken into account is the timing of intercourse with this method because sperm are viable for 48 to 120 hr, and the ovum is viable for 24 hr.
Client Instructions	› Accurately record the number of days in each cycle counting from the first day of menses for a period of at least six cycles. › The start of the fertile period is figured by subtracting 18 days from the number of days in the woman's shortest cycle. › The end of the fertile period is established by subtracting 11 days from the number of days of the longest cycle. For example: » Shortest cycle, 26 – 18 = 8th day » Longest cycle, 30 – 11 = 19th day » Fertile period is days 8 through 19. › Refrain from intercourse during these days to avoid conception.
Advantages	› Most useful when combined with basal body temperature or cervical mucus method. › Inexpensive.
Disadvantages	› Not a very reliable technique. › Requires accurate record-keeping. › Requires compliance in regard to abstinence during fertile periods.
Risks/possible complications/ contraindications	› Various factors can affect and change the time of ovulation and cause unpredictable menstrual cycles. › Risk of pregnancy.

BASAL BODY TEMPERATURE (BBT)	
Definition	› Temperature can drop slightly at the time of ovulation. This can be used to facilitate conception, or be used as a natural contraceptive.
Client Instructions	› A woman is instructed to measure oral temperature prior to getting out of bed each morning to monitor ovulation.
Advantages	› Inexpensive, convenient, and no side effects
Disadvantages	› BBT reliability can be influenced by many variables that can cause inaccurate interpretation of temperature changes, such as stress, fatigue, illness, alcohol, and warmth or coolness of sleeping environment.
Risks/possible complications/ contraindications	› Risk of pregnancy

SYMPTOM-BASED METHOD (CERVICAL MUCUS)	
Definition	› Fertility awareness method based on ovulation. Ovulation occurs approximately 14 days prior to the next menstrual cycle, which is when a woman is fertile. Following ovulation, the cervical mucus becomes thin and flexible under the influence of estrogen and progesterone to allow for sperm viability and motility. The ability for the mucus to stretch between the fingers is greatest during ovulation. This is referred to as the spinnbarkeit sign.
Client Instructions	› Engage in good hand hygiene prior to and following assessment. › Begin examining mucus from the last day of the menstrual cycle. › Mucus is obtained from the vaginal introitus. It is not necessary to reach into the vagina to the cervix. › Do not douche prior to assessment.
Advantages	› A woman can become knowledgeable in recognizing her own mucus characteristics at ovulation, and self-evaluation can be very accurate. › Self-evaluation of cervical mucus also can be diagnostically helpful in determining the start of ovulation while breastfeeding, in noting the commencement of menopause, and in planning a desired pregnancy.
Disadvantages	› Some women can be uncomfortable with touching their genitals and mucus, and therefore will find this method objectionable.
Risks/possible complications/ contraindications	› Assessment of cervical mucus characteristics can be inaccurate if mucus is mixed with semen, blood, contraceptive foams, or discharge from infections. › Risk of pregnancy.

Barrier Methods

CONDOMS	
Definition	› A thin flexible sheath worn on the penis during intercourse to prevent semen from entering the uterus.
Client Instructions	› A man places a condom on his erect penis, leaving an empty space at the tip for a sperm reservoir. › Following ejaculation, a man withdraws his penis from the woman's vagina while holding the rim of the condom to prevent any semen spillage to the woman's vulva or vaginal area. › Can be used in conjunction with spermicidal gel or cream to increase effectiveness.
Advantages	› Protects against STIs, and involves the male in the birth control method.
Disadvantages	› High rate of noncompliance. › Can reduce spontaneity of intercourse. › The penis must be erect to apply a condom. › If the penis is withdrawn while still erect, this can interfere with sexual intercourse.
Risks/possible complications/ contraindications	› Condoms can rupture or leak, thus potentially resulting in an unwanted pregnancy. › Condoms have a one-time usage, which creates a replacement cost. › Condoms made of latex should not be used by those who are sensitive or allergic to latex. › Only water-soluble lubricants should be used with latex condoms to avoid condom breakage.

DIAPHRAGM AND SPERMICIDE	
Definition	› A dome-shaped cup with a flexible rim made of latex or silicone that fits snugly over the cervix with spermicidal cream or gel placed into the dome and around the rim.
Client Instructions	› A female client should be fitted with a diaphragm properly by a provider. › A client must be refitted by the provider every 2 years, if there is a 20% weight fluctuation, any abdominal or pelvic surgery, full-term pregnancy, or second-term abortion. › Requires proper insertion and removal, and the diaphragm should be inspected prior to each time it is used. Prior to coitus, the diaphragm is inserted vaginally over the cervix with spermicidal jelly or cream that is applied to the cervical side of the dome and around the rim. The diaphragm must remain in place for at least 6 hr after coitus. › Spermicide must be reapplied with each act of coitus. › A client should empty her bladder prior to insertion of the diaphragm.
Advantages	› This barrier method eliminates surgery and gives a woman more control over contraception.

DIAPHRAGM AND SPERMICIDE	
Disadvantages	› Diaphragms are inconvenient, interfere with spontaneity, and require reapplication with spermicidal gel, cream, or foam with each act of coitus to be effective. › Requires a prescription and a visit to a provider. › Must be inserted correctly to be effective.
Risks/possible complications/ contraindications	› A diaphragm is not recommended for clients who have a history of toxic shock syndrome (TSS), or frequent, recurrent urinary tract infections. › Increased risk of acquiring TSS. › TSS is caused by a bacterial infection. Indications include high fever, a faint feeling and drop in blood pressure, watery diarrhea, headache, and muscle aches. › Proper hand hygiene, as well as removing diaphragm promptly at 6 hr following coitus, aids in prevention of TSS. › Diaphragms made of latex should not be worn by those who are sensitive or allergic to latex.

Hormonal Methods

MINIPILL	
Definition	› Oral progestins that provide the same action as combined oral contraceptives.
Client Instructions	› A client should take the pill at the same time daily to ensure effectiveness secondary to a low dose of progestin. › A client cannot miss a pill. › A client can need another form of birth control during the first month of use to prevent pregnancy.
Advantages	› The minipill has fewer side effects when compared with a combined oral contraceptive. › Considered safe to take while breastfeeding.
Disadvantages	› Less effective in suppressing ovulation than combined oral contraceptives. › Pill increases occurrence of ovarian cysts. › Pill does not protect against STIs. › Users frequently report breakthrough, irregular, vaginal bleeding, and decreased libido. › Increases appetite
Risks/possible complications/ contraindications	› Oral contraceptive effectiveness decreases when taking medications that affect liver enzymes, such as anticonvulsants and some antibiotics.

COMBINED ORAL CONTRACEPTIVES	
Definition	› Hormonal contraception containing estrogen and progestin, which acts by suppressing ovulation, thickening the cervical mucus to block semen, and altering the uterine decidua to prevent implantation.
Client Instructions	› Medication requires a prescription and follow-up appointments with a provider. › Medication requires consistent and proper use to be effective. › A client is instructed in observing for side effects and danger signs of medication. Signs include chest pain, shortness of breath, leg pain from a possible clot, headache or eye problems from a stroke, or hypertension. › The nurse should instruct the client that if one pill is missed, take one as soon as possible. If two or three pills are missed, instruct the client to follow the manufacturer's instructions. Instruct the client on the use of alternative forms of contraception or abstinence to prevent pregnancy until regular dosing is resumed.
Advantages	› Highly effective if taken correctly and consistently. › Can alleviate dysmenorrhea by decreasing menstrual flow and menstrual cramps. › Reduces acne.
Disadvantages	› Oral contraceptives do not protect against STIs. › Birth control pills can increase the risk of thromboses, breast tenderness, scant or missed menstruation, stroke, nausea, headaches, and hormone-dependent cancers. › Exacerbates conditions affected by fluid retention such as migraines, epilepsy, asthma, kidney, or heart disease.
Risks/possible complications/ contraindications	› Women with a history of blood clots, stroke, cardiac problems, breast or estrogen-related cancers, pregnancy, or smoking (if over 35 years of age), are advised not to take oral contraceptive medications. › Oral contraceptive effectiveness decreases when taking medications that affect liver enzymes, such as anticonvulsants and some antibiotics.

EMERGENCY ORAL CONTRACEPTIVE

Definition	› Morning after pill that prevents fertilization from taking place.
Client Instructions	› Pill is taken within 72 hr after unprotected coitus. › A provider will recommend an over-the-counter antiemetic to be taken 1 hr prior to each dose to counteract the side effects of nausea that can occur with high doses of estrogen and progestin. › Advise a woman to be evaluated for pregnancy if menstruation does not begin within 21 days. › Provide client with counseling about contraception and modification of sexual behaviors that are risky. › Is considered a form of "emergency birth control."
Advantages	› Pill is not taken on a regular basis. › Can be obtained without a prescription by women 17 years and older.
Disadvantages	› Nausea, heavier than normal menstrual bleeding, lower abdominal pain, fatigue, and headache. › Does not provide long-term contraception. › Does not terminate an established pregnancy. › Does not protect against STIs.
Risks/possible complications/ contraindications	› Contraindicated if a client is pregnant or has undiagnosed abnormal vaginal bleeding. › If menstruation does not start within 1 week of expected date, a client can be pregnant.

TRANSDERMAL CONTRACEPTIVE PATCH

Definition	› Contains norelgestromin (progesterone) and ethinyl estradiol, which is delivered at continuous levels through the skin into subcutaneous tissue.
Client Instructions	› A client applies the patch to dry skin overlying subcutaneous tissue of the buttock, abdomen, upper arm, or torso, excluding breast area. › Requires patch replacement once a week. › Patch is applied the same day of the week for 3 weeks with no application of the patch on the fourth week.
Advantages	› Maintains consistent blood levels of hormone. › Avoids liver metabolism of medication because it is not absorbed in the gastrointestinal tract. › Decreases risk of forgetting daily pill.
Disadvantages	› Patch does not protect against STIs. › Poses same side effects as oral contraceptives. › Skin reaction can occur from patch application.
Risks/possible complications/ contraindications	› Same as those of oral contraceptives. › Avoid applying of patch to skin rashes or lesions.

INJECTABLE PROGESTINS (DEPO-PROVERA)

Definition	› An intramuscular injection (a subcutaneous injection is also available) given to a female client every 11 to 13 weeks.
Client Instructions	› Start of injections should be during the first 5 days of a client's menstrual cycle and every 11 to 13 weeks thereafter. Injections in postpartum nonbreastfeeding women should begin within 5 days following delivery. For breastfeeding women, injections should start in the sixth week postpartum. › Advise clients to keep follow-up appointments. › A client should maintain an adequate intake of calcium and vitamin D.
Advantages	› Very effective and requires only four injections per year. › Does not impair lactation.
Disadvantages	› Can prolong amenorrhea. › Irregular or unpredictable bleeding or spotting. › Increases the risk of thromboembolism. › Decreases bone mineral density (loss of calcium). › Does not protect against STIs. › Should only be used as a long-term method of birth control (more than 2 years) if other birth control methods are inadequate.
Risks/possible complications/ contraindications	› Avoid massaging injection site following administration to avoid accelerating medication absorption, which will shorten the duration of its effectiveness.

CONTRACEPTIVE VAGINAL RING (NUVARING)

Definition	› Contains etonogestrel and ethinyl estradiol that is delivered at continuous levels vaginally.
Client Instructions	› A client inserts the ring vaginally. › Requires ring replacement after 3 weeks, and placement of new vaginal ring within 7 days. Insertion should occur on the same day of the week monthly.
Advantages	› Vaginal ring does not have to be fitted. › Decreases the risk of forgetting to take the pill.
Disadvantages	› Vaginal ring does not protect against STIs. › Poses the same side effects as oral contraceptives. › Some clients report discomfort during intercourse.
Risks/possible complications/ contraindications	› Blood clots, hypertension, stroke, heart attack. › Vaginal irritation, increased vaginal secretions, headache, weight gain, and nausea.

IMPLANTABLE PROGESTIN ETONOGESTREL (IMPLANON)

Definition	› Requires a minor surgical procedure to subdermally implant and remove a single rod containing etonogestrel on the inner side of the upper aspect of the arm.
Client Instructions	› Avoid trauma to the area of implantation.
Advantages	› Effective continuous contraception for 3 years. › Reversible. › Can be used by mothers who are breastfeeding after 4 weeks postpartum.
Disadvantages	› Etonogestrel can cause irregular menstrual bleeding. › Etonogestrel does not protect against STIs. › Most common side effect is irregular and unpredictable menstruation. › Headache.
Risks/possible complications/ contraindications	› Increased risk of ectopic pregnancy if pregnancy occurs.

INTRAUTERINE DEVICE (IUD)

Definition	› A chemically active T-shaped device that is inserted through a woman's cervix and placed in the uterus by the provider. Releases a chemical substance that damages sperm in transit to the uterine tubes and prevents fertilization.
Client Instructions	› The device must be monitored monthly by clients after menstruation to ensure the presence of the small string that hangs from the device into the upper part of the vagina to rule out migration or expulsion of the device.
Advantages	› An IUD can maintain effectiveness for 1 to 10 years. 　» The copper IUD is approved for 10 years. 　» The Mirena IUD is approved for up to 5 years. › Contraception can be reversed. › Does not interfere with spontaneity. › Safe for mothers who are breastfeeding. › It is 99% effective in preventing pregnancy.
Disadvantages	› An IUD can increase the risk of pelvic inflammatory disease, uterine perforation, or ectopic pregnancy. › A client should report to the provider late or abnormal spotting or bleeding, abdominal pain or pain with intercourse, abnormal or foul-smelling vaginal discharge, fever, chills, a change in string length, or if IUD cannot be located. › An IUD does not protect from STIs.
Risks/possible complications/ contraindications	› Best used by women in a monogamous relationship due to the risks of STIs. › Can cause irregular menstrual bleeding. › A risk of bacterial vaginosis, uterine perforation, or uterine expulsion. › Must be removed in the event of pregnancy.

Transcervical Sterilization

ESSURE	
Definition	› Insertion of small flexible agents through the vagina and cervix into the fallopian tubes. This results in the development of scar tissue in the tubes preventing conception. › Examination must be done after 3 months to ensure fallopian tubes are blocked.
Client Instruction	› Normal activities can be resumed by most clients within 1 day of the procedure.
Advantages	› Quick procedure that requires no general anesthesia. › Nonhormonal means of birth control. › Essure is 99.8% effective in preventing pregnancy. › Rapid return to normal activities of daily living.
Disadvantages	› Not reversible. › Not intended for use in the client who is postpartum. › Delay in effectiveness for 3 months. Therefore, an alternative means of birth control should be used until confirmation of blocked fallopian tubes occurs. › Changes in menstrual patterns.
Risks/possible complications/ contraindications	› Perforation can occur › Unwanted pregnancy can occur if a client has unprotected sexual intercourse during the first 3 months following the procedure. › Increased risk of ectopic pregnancy if pregnancy occurs.

Surgical Methods

FEMALE STERILIZATION (BILATERAL TUBAL LIGATION SALPINGECTOMY)	
Definition	› A surgical procedure consisting of severance and/or burning or blocking the fallopian tubes to prevent fertilization.
Procedure	› The cutting, burning, or blocking of the fallopian tubes to prevent the ovum from being fertilized by the sperm.
Advantages	› Permanent contraception. › Sexual function is unaffected.
Disadvantages	› A surgical procedure carrying risks related to anesthesia, complications, infection, hemorrhage, or trauma. › Considered irreversible in the event that a client desires conception.
Risks/possible complications/ contraindications	› Risk of ectopic pregnancy if pregnancy occurs.

MALE STERILIZATION (VASECTOMY)

Definition	› A surgical procedure consisting of ligation and severance of the vas deferens.
Procedure	› The cutting of the vas deferens in the male as a form of permanent sterilization. Reinforce the need for alternate forms of birth control for approximately 20 ejaculations or 1 week to several months to allow all of the sperm to clear the vas deferens. This will ensure complete male infertility.
Client Instruction	› Following the procedure, scrotal support and moderate activity for a couple of days is recommended to reduce discomfort. › Sterility is delayed until the proximal portion of the vas deferens is cleared of all remaining sperm (approximately 20 ejaculations). › Alternate forms of birth control must be used until the vas deferens is cleared of sperm. › Follow up is important for sperm count.
Advantages	› A vasectomy is a permanent contraceptive method. › Procedure is short, safe, and simple. › Sexual function is not impaired.
Disadvantages	› Requires surgery. › Considered irreversible in the event that a client desires conception.
Risks/ possible complications/ contraindications	› Complications are rare, but can include bleeding, infection, and anesthesia reaction.

View Images
› Bilateral Tubal Ligation   › Vasectomy

APPLICATION EXERCISES

1. A nurse in a health clinic is reviewing contraceptive use with a group of adolescent clients. Which of the following statements by an adolescent requires clarification?

    A. "A water-soluble lubricant should be used with condoms."

    B. "Spermicide is applied once when using a diaphragm."

    C. "Oral contraceptives can improve a case of acne."

    D. "A contraceptive patch is worn for a week."

2. A nurse is reviewing instructions with a client who has been prescribed oral contraceptives about danger signs. The nurse evaluates that the client understands the teaching regarding side effects when she states the need to report which of the following?

    A. Reduced menstrual flow or amenorrhea

    B. Weight gain or breast tenderness

    C. Chest pain or shortness of breath

    D. Mild hypertension or headaches

3. A nurse in an obstetrical clinic is reinforcing education about contraception to a 21-year-old client. Which of the following statements by the client requesting information regarding an IUD indicates a need for additional teaching?

    A. "An IUD may increase my risk for an ectopic pregnancy."

    B. "I will wait until I have a child before I can have an IUD."

    C. "I might have irregular bleeding after I get an IUD."

    D. "A change in the string length of my IUD is expected."

4. A nurse in a clinic is reinforcing teaching with a client about her new prescription for medroxyprogesterone (Depo-Provera). Which of the following should be included in the teaching?

    A. "Weight loss can occur."

    B. "You are protected against STIs."

    C. "You should be taking calcium also."

    D. "You should avoid taking antibiotics when using this contraceptive."

5. Which of the following should the nurse include when reinforcing teaching with a client about the potential disadvantages of the minipill? (Select all that apply.)

_____ A. Amenorrhea

_____ B. Irregular vaginal bleeding

_____ C. Increased appetite

_____ D. Decreased libido

_____ E. Ovarian cysts

6. A nurse is reviewing teaching with a male client who is considering a vasectomy. Which of the following should be included in the review of the teaching? Use the ATI Active Learning Template: Basic Concept to complete this item to include the following sections:

A. Topic Descriptor: Define the procedure.

B. Related Content: Describe one advantage and one disadvantage of this form of contraception.

C. Underlying Principles: Describe two teaching points for this client.

APPLICATION EXERCISES KEY

1. A. INCORRECT: The client should use water-soluble lubricants when using a condom.

    B. **CORRECT:** With each act of coitus, the client should apply a spermicide.

    C. INCORRECT: Clients who take oral contraceptives can have reduced acne.

    D. INCORRECT: The client should replace the contraceptive patch once a week.

    Ⓝ NCLEX® Connection: Health Promotion and Maintenance, Lifestyle Choices

2. A. INCORRECT: Reduced menstrual flow, or amenorrhea, is a common side effect of oral contraceptives and usually subsides after a few months of use.

    B. INCORRECT: Weight gain or breast tenderness is a common side effect of oral contraceptives and usually subsides after a few months of use.

    C. **CORRECT:** Chest pain or shortness of breath can indicate a pulmonary embolus or myocardial infarction.

    D. INCORRECT: Mild hypertension or headaches are a common side effect of oral contraceptives and usually subside after a few months of use.

    Ⓝ NCLEX® Connection: Health Promotion and Maintenance, Lifestyle Choices

3. A. INCORRECT: An IUD can increase the risk for an ectopic pregnancy.

    B. INCORRECT: Clients should have at least one child to be a candidate for an IUD.

    C. INCORRECT: An IUD can cause irregular vaginal bleeding.

    D. **CORRECT:** A client should report to the provider a change in the length of the string of an IUD because it can indicate expulsion.

    Ⓝ NCLEX® Connection: Health Promotion and Maintenance, Lifestyle Choices

4. A. INCORRECT: Weight gain can occur.

    B. INCORRECT: Depo-Provera does not provide protection against STIs.

    C. **CORRECT:** Clients should take calcium and vitamin D to prevent loss of bone density, which can occur when taking Depo-Provera.

    D. INCORRECT: Antibiotics are not contraindicated when taking Depo-Provera.

    Ⓝ NCLEX® Connection: Health Promotion and Maintenance, Lifestyle Choices

5. A. INCORRECT: Amenorrhea is not a disadvantage of the minipill.

    B. **CORRECT:** Irregular vaginal bleeding is a disadvantage of the minipill.

    C. **CORRECT:** Increased appetite is a disadvantage of the minipill.

    D. **CORRECT:** Decreased libido is a disadvantage of the minipill.

    E. **CORRECT:** A disadvantage of the minipill is the increased occurrence of ovarian cysts.

    (N) NCLEX® Connection: Health Promotion and Maintenance, Lifestyle Choices

6. *Using the ATI Active Learning: Basic Concept*

    A. Topic Descriptor
        • Surgical procedure involving ligation and severance of the vas deferens.

    B. Related Content
        • Advantages
            ○ A permanent contraceptive method
            ○ Procedure is short, safe, and simple
            ○ Sexual function is not impaired
        • Disadvantages
            ○ A surgical procedure; considered irreversible.

    C. Underlying Principles
        • Scrotal support and moderate activity are recommended for several days after the procedure to improve comfort.
        • An alternate form of contraception should be used for approximately 20 ejaculations to ensure that the vas deferens is cleared of remaining sperm.
        • A follow-up sperm count should be done.

    (N) NCLEX® Connection: Health Promotion and Maintenance, Lifestyle Choices

chapter 2

Overview

- Recognizing changes during pregnancy is helpful for both clients and nurses. The nurse and provider assess findings during the client's initial prenatal visit.
- Signs of pregnancy are classified into three groups.
  - Presumptive
  - Probable
  - Positive
- Calculating delivery date, determining number of pregnancies, and evaluating physiological status of a client who is pregnant are performed.

Signs of Pregnancy

- Presumptive signs – changes that the woman experiences that make her think that she might be pregnant. These changes can be subjective symptoms or objective signs. Signs also can be a result of physiological factors other than pregnancy (peristalsis, infections, and stress).
  - Amenorrhea
  - Fatigue
  - Nausea and vomiting
  - Urinary frequency
  - Breast changes – darkened areolae, enlarged Montgomery's glands
  - Quickening – slight fluttering movements of the fetus felt by a woman, usually between 16 to 20 weeks of gestation
- Probable signs – changes that make the examiner suspect a woman is pregnant (primarily related to physical changes of the uterus). Signs can be caused by physiological factors other than pregnancy (pelvic congestion, tumors).
  - Abdominal enlargement related to changes in uterine size, shape, and position
  - Hegar's sign – softening and compressibility of lower uterus
  - Chadwick's sign – deepened violet-bluish color of cervix and vaginal mucosa
  - Goodell's sign – softening of cervical tip
  - Ballottement – rebound of unengaged fetus
  - Braxton Hicks contractions – false contractions; painless, irregular, and usually relieved by walking
  - Positive pregnancy test
  - Fetal outline felt by examiner
- Positive signs – signs that can be explained only by pregnancy.
  - Fetal heart sounds
  - Visualization of fetus by ultrasound
  - Fetal movement palpated by an experienced examiner

Verifying Possible Pregnancy Using Serum and Urine Pregnancy Testing

- Serum and urine tests provide an accurate assessment for the presence of human chorionic gonadotropin (hCG). hCG production can start as early as the day of implantation and can be detected as early as 8 to 10 days after conception.

- Production of hCG begins with implantation, peaks at about 50 to 70 days of gestation, declines until around 80 days of pregnancy, and then gradually increases until term.

- Higher levels of hCG can indicate multifetal pregnancy, ectopic pregnancy, hydatidiform mole (gestational trophoblastic disease), or a genetic abnormality such as Down syndrome. Lower blood levels of hCG can suggest a miscarriage.

- Some medications (anticonvulsants, diuretics, tranquilizers) can cause false-positive or false-negative pregnancy results.

- Urine samples should be first-voided morning specimens.

Calculating Delivery Date and Determining Number of Pregnancies for Pregnant Client

- Naegele's rule – Take the first day of the woman's last menstrual cycle, subtract 3 months, and then add 7 days and 1 year, adjusting for the year as necessary.

- Measurement of fundal height in centimeters from the symphysis pubis to the top of the uterine fundus (between 18 and 32 weeks of gestation).
  - ○ Approximates the gestational age

- Gravidity – number of pregnancies.
  - ○ Nulligravida – a woman who has never been pregnant
  - ○ Primigravida – a woman in her first pregnancy
  - ○ Multigravida – a woman who has had two or more pregnancies
  - ○ Parity – number of pregnancies in which the fetus or fetuses reach viability (approximately 20 weeks) regardless of whether the fetus is born alive
    - ▪ Nullipara – no pregnancy beyond the stage of viability
    - ▪ Primipara – has completed one pregnancy to stage of viability
    - ▪ Multipara – has completed two or more pregnancies to stage of viability

- GTPAL acronym
  - ○ Gravidity
  - ○ Term births (38 weeks or more)
  - ○ Preterm births (from viability up to 37 weeks)
  - ○ Abortions/miscarriages (prior to viability)
  - ○ Living children

Physiological Status of Pregnant Client

- Reproductive – Uterus increases in size and changes shape and position. Ovulation and menses cease during pregnancy.

- Cardiovascular – Cardiac output and blood volume increase (45% to 50% at term) to meet the greater metabolic needs. Heart rate increases during pregnancy.

- Respiratory – Maternal oxygen needs increase. During the last trimester, the size of the chest can enlarge, allowing for lung expansion, as the uterus pushes upward. Respiratory rate increases and total lung capacity decreases.

- Musculoskeletal – Body alterations and weight increase necessitate an adjustment in posture. Pelvic joints relax.

- Gastrointestinal – Nausea and vomiting can occur due to hormonal changes and/or an increase of pressure within the abdominal cavity as the pregnant client's stomach and intestines are displaced within the abdomen. Constipation can occur due to increased transit time of food through the gastrointestinal tract, and thus, increased water absorption.

- Renal – Filtration rate increases secondary to the influence of pregnancy hormones and an increase in blood volume and metabolic demands. The amount of urine produced remains the same. Urinary frequency is common during pregnancy.

- Endocrine – The placenta becomes an endocrine organ that produces large amounts of hCG, progesterone, estrogen, human placental lactogen, and prostaglandins. Hormones are very active during pregnancy and function to maintain pregnancy and prepare the body for delivery.

- Body Image Changes

  ○ Due to physical and psychological changes that occur, the pregnant woman requires support from her provider and family members.

  ○ In the first trimester of pregnancy, physiological changes are not obvious. Many women look forward to the changes so that pregnancy will be more noticeable.

  ○ During the second trimester, there are rapid physical changes due to the enlargement of the abdomen and breasts. Skin changes also occur, such as stretch marks and hyperpigmentation. These changes can affect a woman's mobility. She can find herself losing her balance and feeling back or leg discomfort and fatigue. These factors can lead to a negative body image. The client can make statements of resentment toward the pregnancy and express anxiousness for the pregnancy to be over soon.

- Expected Vital Signs

  ○ Blood pressure measurements are within the prepregnancy range during the first trimester.

  ○ Blood pressure decreases 5 to 10 mm Hg for both the diastolic and the systolic during the second trimester.

  ○ Blood pressure should return to the prepregnancy baseline range after approximately 20 weeks of gestation.

  ○ Position of the pregnant woman also can affect blood pressure. In the supine position, blood pressure can appear to be lower due to the weight and pressure of the gravid uterus on the vena cava, which decreases venous blood flow to the heart. Maternal hypotension and fetal hypoxia can occur, which is referred to as supine hypotensive syndrome or supine vena cava syndrome. Manifestations include dizziness, lightheadedness, and pale, clammy skin. Encourage the client to engage in maternal positioning on the left-lateral side, semi-Fowler's position, or, if supine, with a wedge placed under one hip to alleviate pressure to the vena cava.

○ Pulse increases 10 to 15/min around 20 weeks of gestation and remains elevated throughout the remainder of the pregnancy.

○ Respirations increase by 1 to 2/min. Respiratory changes in pregnancy are attributed to the elevation of the diaphragm by as much as 4 cm, as well as changes to the chest wall to facilitate increased maternal oxygen demands. Some shortness of breath can be noted.

• Expected Physical Assessment Findings

○ Fetal heart tones are heard at a normal baseline rate of 110 to 160/min with reassuring FHR accelerations noted, which indicates an intact fetal CNS.

○ The client's heart changes in size and shape with resulting cardiac hypertrophy to accommodate increased blood volume and increased cardiac output. Heart sounds also change to accommodate the increase in blood volume with a more distinguishable splitting of S_1 and S_2, with S_3 more easily heard following 20 weeks of gestation. Murmurs also can be auscultated. Heart size and shape should return to normal shortly after delivery.

○ Uterine size changes from a uterine weight of 50 to 1,000 g (0.1 to 2.2 lb). By 36 weeks of gestation, the top of the uterus and the fundus will reach the xiphoid process. This can cause the pregnant woman to experience shortness of breath as the uterus pushes against the diaphragm.

○ Cervical changes are obvious as a purplish-blue color extends into the vagina and labia, and the cervix becomes markedly soft.

○ Breast changes occur due to hormones of pregnancy, with the breasts increasing in size and the areolas darkening.

○ Skin changes

▪ Chloasma – Pigmentation increases on the face.

▪ Linea nigra – Dark line of pigmentation from the umbilicus extending to the pubic area.

▪ Striae gravidarum – Stretch marks most notably found on the abdomen, breasts, and thighs.

Nursing Interventions for the Pregnant Client

• Acknowledge the client's concerns about pregnancy, and encourage sharing of these feelings while providing an atmosphere free of judgment.

• Discuss with the client the expected physiological changes and a possible timeline for a return to the prepregnant state.

• Assist the client in setting goals for the postpartum period in regard to self-care and newborn care.

• Refer the client to counseling if body image concerns appear to have a negative impact on the pregnancy.

• Reinforce education about the expected physiological and psychosocial changes. Common discomforts of pregnancy and ways to resolve those discomforts are reviewed during prenatal visits.

• Encourage the client to keep all follow-up appointments and to contact the provider immediately if there is any bleeding, leakage of fluid, or contractions at any time during the pregnancy.

APPLICATION EXERCISES

1. A nurse is caring for a client who is pregnant and states that her last menstrual period was April 1, 2013. Which of the following is the client's estimated date of delivery?

    A. Jan. 8, 2014

    B. Jan. 15, 2014

    C. Feb. 8, 2014

    D. Feb. 15, 2014

2. A nurse in a prenatal clinic is caring for a client who is in the first trimester of pregnancy. The client's health record includes this data: G3 T1 P0 A1 L1. How should the nurse interpret this information? (Select all that apply.)

    _____ A. Client has delivered one newborn at term.

    _____ B. Client has experienced no preterm labor.

    _____ C. Client has been through active labor.

    _____ D. Client has had two prior pregnancies.

    _____ E. Client has one living child.

3. A nurse is reviewing the health record of a client who is pregnant. The provider indicated the client exhibits probable signs of pregnancy. Which of the following would be included? (Select all that apply.)

    _____ A. Montgomery's glands

    _____ B. Goodell's sign

    _____ C. Ballottement

    _____ D. Chadwick's sign

    _____ E. Quickening

4. A nurse in a prenatal clinic is caring for a client who is pregnant and experiencing episodes of maternal hypotension. The client asks the nurse what causes these episodes. Which of the following is an appropriate response by the nurse?

    A. "This is due to an increase in blood volume."

    B. "This is due to pressure from the uterus on the diaphragm."

    C. "This is due to the weight of the uterus on the vena cava."

    D. "This is due to increased cardiac output."

5. A nurse in a clinic receives a phone call from a client who believes she is pregnant and would like to be tested in the clinic to confirm her pregnancy. Which of the following information should the nurse provide to the client?

    A. "You should wait until 4 weeks after conception to be tested."

    B. "You should be off any medications for 24 hours prior to the test."

    C. "You should be NPO for at least 8 hours prior to the test."

    D. "You should collect urine from the first morning void."

6. A nurse is caring for a client who is in the fourth week of gestation. The client asks about skin and breast changes that can occur during pregnancy. What is an appropriate response by the nurse? Use the ATI Active Learning Template: Basic Concept to complete this item to include the following:

    A. Related Content: Describe at least three changes that occur to skin and breasts during pregnancy.

    B. Underlying Principles: Describe the basis for these changes.

APPLICATION EXERCISES KEY

1. A. **CORRECT:** April 1, 2013, minus 3 months, plus 7 days and 1 year equals an estimated date of delivery of Jan. 8, 2014.

    B. INCORRECT: This date is incorrect using Naegele's rule.

    C. INCORRECT: This date is incorrect using Naegele's rule.

    D. INCORRECT: This date is incorrect using Naegele's rule.

    Ⓝ NCLEX® Connection: Health Promotion and Maintenance, Data Collection Techniques

2. A. **CORRECT:** T1 indicates the client has delivered one newborn at term.

    B. INCORRECT: P0 indicates the client has had no preterm deliveries.

    C. INCORRECT: A1 indicates the client has had one miscarriage.

    D. **CORRECT:** G3 indicates the client has had two prior pregnancies and is currently pregnant.

    E. **CORRECT:** L1 indicates the client has one living child.

    Ⓝ NCLEX® Connection: Health Promotion and Maintenance, Data Collection Techniques

3. A. INCORRECT: Montgomery's glands are a presumptive sign of pregnancy.

    B. **CORRECT:** Goodell's sign is a probable sign of pregnancy.

    C. **CORRECT:** Ballottement is a probable sign of pregnancy.

    D. **CORRECT:** Chadwick's sign is a probable sign of pregnancy.

    E. INCORRECT: Quickening is a presumptive sign of pregnancy.

    Ⓝ NCLEX® Connection: Health Promotion and Maintenance, Data Collection Techniques

4.   A. INCORRECT: An increase in blood volume during pregnancy results in cardiac hypertrophy.

    B. INCORRECT: Pressure from the gravid uterus on the diaphragm can cause the client to experience shortness of breath.

    C. **CORRECT:** Maternal hypotension occurs when the client is lying in the supine position, and the weight of the gravid uterus places pressure on the vena cava, decreasing venous blood flow to the heart.

    D. INCORRECT: An increase in cardiac output during pregnancy results in cardiac hypertrophy.

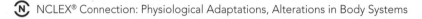 NCLEX® Connection: Physiological Adaptations, Alterations in Body Systems

5.   A. INCORRECT: The production of hCG can be detected as early as 8 to 10 days after conception.

    B. INCORRECT: Clients are not advised to stop taking medications in preparation for pregnancy tests. Medications should be reviewed to determine whether they can affect the results.

    C. INCORRECT: Clients are not advised to remain NPO prior to pregnancy testing. Serum or blood tests are not affected by food or fluid intake.

    D. **CORRECT:** Urine pregnancy tests should be done on a first-voided morning specimen to provide the most accurate results.

NCLEX® Connection: Reduction of Risk Potential, Diagnostic Tests

6. *Using the ATI Active Learning Template: Basic Concept*

    A. Related Content
- Skin changes: hyperpigmentation; linea nigra; chloasma (mask of pregnancy) on the face; striae gravidarum (stretch marks), most pronounced on abdomen, breasts, and thighs
- Breast changes: darkening of the areola, enlarged Montgomery's glands, increase in size and heaviness, increased sensitivity

    B. Underlying Principles
- Increase in estrogen and progesterone occurring during pregnancy

NCLEX® Connection: Physiological Adaptations, Alterations in Body Systems

chapter **3**

Overview

- Prenatal care involves nursing assessments and client education for expectant mothers. When providing prenatal care, nurses must take into account cultural considerations.

- Prenatal education encompasses information provided to a client who is pregnant. Major areas of focus include assisting the client in self-care of the discomforts of pregnancy, promoting a safe outcome to pregnancy, and fostering positive feelings by the pregnant woman and her family regarding the childbearing experience.

- Prenatal care dramatically reduces infant and maternal morbidity and mortality rates by early detection and treatment of potential problems. A majority of birth defects occur between 2 and 8 weeks of gestation.

Nursing Assessments

- Nurses play an integral role in determining a client's current knowledge, previous pregnancies, and birthing experiences.

- Data collection in prenatal care includes obtaining information regarding:

  - Reproductive and obstetrical history (contraception use, gynecological diagnoses, and obstetrical difficulties).

  - Medical history, including the woman's immune status (rubella and hepatitis B).

  - Family history, such as genetic disorders.

  - Any recent or current illnesses or infections.

  - Current medications, including use of herbal preparations, substance use, and alcohol consumption. The nurse should display a nonjudgmental, matter-of-fact demeanor when interviewing a client regarding substance abuse, and observe for indications such as lack of grooming.

  - Psychosocial history (a client's emotional response to pregnancy, adolescent pregnancy, spouse, support system, history of depression, domestic violence issues).

  - Any hazardous environmental exposures; current work conditions.

  - Current exercise and diet habits as well as lifestyle.

- Ascertain what a client's goals are for the birthing process. Discuss birthing methods, such as Lamaze, and pain control options (epidural, natural childbirth).

- Prenatal care begins with an initial prenatal visit and continues throughout pregnancy. In an uneventful pregnancy, prenatal visits are scheduled monthly for 7 months, every 2 weeks during the eighth month, and every week during the last month.
  - At the initial prenatal visit
    - Determine estimated date of birth based on the last menstrual period.
    - Assist with obtaining medical and nursing history to include social supports, and review of systems (to assist with determining risk factors).
    - Perform data collection to include a client's baseline weight, vital signs, and assist with pelvic examination. Identify signs and symptoms of urinary tract infections (UTIs) and kidney infection.
    - Review initial laboratory tests.
  - Ongoing prenatal visits
    - Monitoring weight, blood pressure, and urine for glucose, protein, and leukocytes.
    - Monitoring for the presence of edema.
    - Monitoring fetal development.
      - FHR can be heard by Doppler at 10 to 12 weeks of gestation or heard with an ultrasound stethoscope at 16 to 20 weeks of gestation. Listen at the midline, right above the symphysis pubis, by holding the stethoscope firmly on the abdomen.
      - Assist with measuring fundal height after 12 weeks of gestation.

 View Video: Measuring Fundal Height

      - Monitor for fetal movement between 16 and 20 weeks of gestation.
    - Providing instructions for self-care to include management of common discomforts and concerns of pregnancy (nausea and vomiting, fatigue, backache, varicosities, heartburn, activity, sexuality).

PRENATAL CARE: ROUTINE LABORATORY TESTS
Blood type, Rh factor, and presence of irregular antibodies
› Determines the risk for maternal-fetal blood incompatibility (erythroblastosis fetalis) or neonatal hyperbilirubinemia. Indirect Coombs test identifies clients sensitized to Rh-positive blood. For clients who are Rh-negative and not sensitized, the indirect Coombs test is repeated between 24 and 28 weeks of gestation.
CBC with differential, Hgb, and Hct
› Detects infection and anemia.
Hgb electrophoresis
› Identifies hemoglobinopathies (sickle cell anemia and thalassemia).
Rubella titer
› Determines immunity to rubella.
Hepatitis B screen
› Identifies carriers of hepatitis B.

PRENATAL CARE: ROUTINE LABORATORY TESTS

Group B streptococcus (GBS)

› Obtained at 35 to 37 weeks of gestation.

Urinalysis with microscopic examination of pH, specific gravity, color, sediment, protein, glucose, albumin, RBCs, WBCs, casts, acetone, and human chorionic gonadotropin (hCG)

› Identifies pregnancy, diabetes mellitus, gestational hypertension, renal disease, and infection.

One-hour glucose tolerance (oral ingestion or IV administration of concentrated glucose with venous sample taken 1 hr later [fasting not necessary])

› Identifies hyperglycemia; done at initial visit for at-risk clients, and at 24 to 28 weeks of gestation for all pregnant women (greater than 140 mg/dL requires follow up).

Three-hour glucose tolerance (fasting overnight prior to oral ingestion or IV administration of concentrated glucose with a venous sample taken 1, 2, and 3 hr later)

› Used in clients who have elevated 1-hr glucose test as a screening tool for diabetes mellitus. A diagnosis of gestational diabetes requires two elevated blood-glucose readings.

Papanicolaou (Pap) test

› Screening tool for cervical cancer, herpes simplex type 2, and/or human papillomavirus.

Vaginal/cervical culture

› Detects streptococcus ß-hemolytic, bacterial vaginosis, or sexually transmitted infections (gonorrhea and chlamydia).

PPD (tuberculosis screening), chest x-ray after 20 weeks of gestation with PPD test

› Identifies exposure to tuberculosis.

Venereal disease research laboratory (VDRL)

› Syphilis screening mandated by law.

HIV

› Detects HIV infection (the Centers for Disease Control and Prevention and the American Congress of Obstetricians and Gynecologists recommend testing all clients who are pregnant unless the client refuses testing).

Toxoplasmosis, other infections, rubella, cytomegalovirus, and herpes virus (TORCH) screening when indicated

› Screening for a group of infections capable of crossing the placenta and adversely affecting fetal development.

Maternal serum alpha-fetoprotein (MSAFP)

› Screening occurs between 15 to 22 weeks of gestation. Used to rule out Down syndrome (low level) and neural tube defects (high level). Instead of the MSAFP, the provider can decide to use a more reliable indicator and opt for the "quad screen" at 16 to 18 weeks of gestation. This includes AFP, inhibin-A, a combination analysis of human chorionic gonadotropin, and estriol.

○ Assist with Leopold maneuvers to palpate presentation and position of the fetus.

○ Assist the provider with the gynecological examination. This examination is performed to determine the status of a client's reproductive organs and birth canal. Pelvic measurements determine whether the pelvis will allow for the passage of the fetus at delivery.

  ▪ Have the client empty her bladder and take deep breaths during the examination to decrease discomfort.

○ Administer Rho(D) immune globulin (RhoGAM) IM around 28 weeks of gestation for clients who are Rh-negative. *— 72 hrs — within After giving birthday*

Client Education

- Prenatal education includes health promotion, preparation for pregnancy and birth, common discomforts of pregnancy, and warning/danger signs to report.

- Health Promotion

  ○ Preconception and prenatal education emphasizes healthy behaviors that promote the health of the pregnant woman and her fetus.

    ▪ A client is instructed to avoid all over-the-counter medications, supplements, and prescription medications unless the provider who is supervising her care has knowledge of this practice.

    ▪ Alcohol (birth defects) and tobacco (low birth weight) are contraindicated during pregnancy.

    ▪ Substance use of any kind is to be avoided during pregnancy and lactation. Strategies to reduce or eliminate substance use are reviewed.

  ○ Instruct a client about the following.

    ▪ Need for flu immunization

    ▪ Smoking cessation

    ▪ Treatment of current infections

    ▪ Genetic testing and counseling

    ▪ Exposure to hazardous materials

  ○ Exercise during pregnancy yields positive benefits and should consist of 30 min of moderate exercise (walking or swimming) daily if not medically or obstetrically contraindicated.

    ▪ Avoid the use of hot tubs or saunas.

    ▪ Consume at least 2 to 3 L of water each day from food and beverage sources.

- Preparation for Pregnancy and Birth

  ○ Nurses provide anticipatory instructions to the pregnant client and her family about the following.

    ▪ Physical and emotional changes during pregnancy and interventions that can be implemented to provide relief

    ▪ Signs and symptoms of complications to report to the provider

    ▪ Birthing options available to enhance the birthing process

- Maternal adaptation to pregnancy and the attainment of the maternal role – whereby the idea of pregnancy is accepted and assimilated into the client's way of life – includes hormonal and psychological aspects.

  - Emotional lability is experienced by many women with unpredictable mood changes and increased irritability, tearfulness, and anger alternating with feelings of joy and cheerfulness. This can result from hormonal changes.

  - A feeling of ambivalence about the pregnancy, which is a normal response, can occur early in the pregnancy and resolve before the third trimester. It consists of conflicting feelings (joy, pleasure, sorrow, hostility) about the pregnancy. These feelings can occur simultaneously, whether the pregnancy was planned or not.

- The nurse anticipates reviewing prenatal instruction topics with a client based on her current knowledge and previous pregnancy and birth experiences. The client's readiness to learn is enhanced when the nurse provides instructions during the appropriate trimester based on learning needs. Using a variety of educational methods, such as pamphlets and videos, and having the client verbalize and demonstrate learned topics will ensure that learning has taken place.

  - First Trimester

    - Physical and psychosocial changes

    - Common discomforts of pregnancy and measures to provide relief

    - Lifestyle: exercise, stress, nutrition, sexual health, dental care, over-the-counter and prescription medications, tobacco, alcohol, substance use, and STIs (encourage safe sexual practices)

    - Possible complications and signs to report (preterm labor)

    - Fetal growth and development

    - Prenatal exercise

    - Expected laboratory testing

  - Second Trimester

    - Benefits of breastfeeding

    - Common discomforts and relief measures

    - Lifestyle: sex and pregnancy, rest and relaxation, posture, body mechanics, clothing, and seat belt safety and travel

    - Fetal movement

    - Complications (preterm labor, gestational hypertension, gestational diabetes mellitus, premature rupture of membranes)

    - Preparation for childbirth and childbirth education classes

    - Review of birthing methods

    - Development of a birth plan (verbal or written agreement about what client wishes during labor and delivery)

  - Third Trimester

    - Childbirth preparation

      ‣ Childbirth classes or birth plan

      ‣ Breathing and relaxation techniques

      ‣ Use of effleurage and counterpressure

- ‣ Application of heat/cold, touch and massage, and water therapy

- ‣ Use of transcutaneous electrical nerve stimulation (TENS)

- ‣ Acupressure and acupuncture

- ‣ Music and aromatherapy

- ‣ Discussion regarding pain management during labor and birth (natural childbirth, epidural)

- ‣ Manifestations of preterm labor and labor

- ‣ Labor process

- ‣ Infant care

- ‣ Postpartum care

- ▫ Fetal movement/kick counts to ascertain fetal well-being. A client should be instructed to count and record fetal movements or kicks daily.

  - ‣ Mothers should count fetal activity two or three times a day for 60 min each time. Fetal movements of less than 3/hr or movements that cease entirely for 12 hr indicate a need for further evaluation.

- ▫ Diagnostic testing for fetal well-being (nonstress test, biophysical profile, ultrasound, and contraction stress test).

- • Common Discomforts of Pregnancy

  - ○ Nausea and vomiting can occur during the first trimester. The client should eat crackers or dry toast 30 min to 1 hr before rising in the morning to relieve discomfort. Instruct the client to avoid having an empty stomach and ingesting spicy, greasy, or gas-forming foods. Encourage the client to drink fluids between meals.

  - ○ Breast tenderness can occur during the first trimester. The client should wear a bra that provides adequate support.

  - ○ Urinary frequency can occur during the first and third trimesters. The client should empty her bladder frequently, decrease fluid intake before bedtime, and use perineal pads. Reinforce teaching on how to perform Kegel exercises (alternate tightening and relaxation of pubococcygeal muscles) to reduce stress incontinence (leakage of urine with coughing and sneezing).

  - ○ Urinary tract infections (UTIs) are common during pregnancy because of renal changes and the vaginal flora becoming more alkaline.

    - ▪ UTI risks can be decreased by encouraging the client to wipe the perineal area from front to back after voiding, avoid bubble baths, wear cotton underpants, avoid tight-fitting pants, and consume plenty of water (8 glasses per day).

    - ▪ Advise the client to urinate before and after intercourse to flush bacteria from the urethra that are present or introduced during intercourse.

    - ▪ Advise the client to urinate as soon as the urge occurs because retaining urine provides an environment for bacterial growth.

    - ▪ Advise the client to notify her provider if her urine is foul-smelling, contains blood, or appears cloudy.

○ Fatigue can occur during the first and third trimesters. Encourage the client to engage in frequent rest periods.

○ Heartburn can occur during the second and third trimesters due to the stomach being displaced by the enlarging uterus and a slowing of gastrointestinal tract motility and digestion brought about by increased progesterone levels. The client should eat small frequent meals, not allow the stomach to get too empty or too full, sit up for 30 min after meals, and check with her provider prior to using any over-the-counter antacids.

○ Constipation can occur during the second and third trimesters. Encourage the client to drink plenty of fluids, eat a diet high in fiber, and exercise regularly.

○ Hemorrhoids can occur during the second and third trimesters. A warm sitz bath, witch hazel pads, and application of topical ointments will help relieve discomfort.

○ Backaches are common during the second and third trimesters. The client is encouraged to exercise regularly, perform pelvic tilt exercises (alternately arching and straightening the back), use proper body mechanics by using the legs to lift rather than the back, and use the side-lying position.

○ Shortness of breath and dyspnea can occur because of the enlarged uterus, which limits inspiration. The client should maintain good posture, sleep with extra pillows, and contact her provider if symptoms worsen.

○ Leg cramps during the third trimester can occur due to the compression of lower-extremity nerves and blood vessels by the enlarging uterus. This can result in poor peripheral circulation as well as an imbalance in the calcium/phosphorus ratio. The client should extend the affected leg, keeping the knee straight, and dorsiflex the foot (toes toward head). Application of heat over the affected muscle or a foot massage while the leg is extended can help relieve cramping. The client should notify her provider if frequent cramping occurs.

○ Varicose veins and lower-extremity edema can occur during the second and third trimesters. The client should rest with her legs elevated, avoid constricting clothing, wear support hose, avoid sitting or standing in one position for extended periods of time, and not sit with her legs crossed at the knees. She should sleep in the left-lateral position and exercise moderately with frequent walking to stimulate venous return.

○ Gingivitis, nasal stuffiness, and epistaxis (nosebleed) can occur as a result of elevated estrogen levels causing increased vascularity and proliferation of connective tissue. The client should gently brush her teeth, observe good dental hygiene, use a humidifier, and use normal saline nose drops or spray.

○ Braxton Hicks contractions, which occur from the first trimester onward, can increase in intensity and frequency during the third trimester. Inform the client that a change of position and walking should cause contractions to subside. If contractions increase in intensity and frequency (true contractions) with regularity, the client should notify her provider.

○ Supine hypotension occurs when a woman lies on her back, and the weight of the gravid uterus compresses her vena cava. This reduces blood supply to the fetus. The client can experience feelings of lightheadedness and faintness. Instruct the client to lie in a side-lying or semi-sitting position with her knees slightly flexed.

- Danger Signs During Pregnancy
  - The following indicate potential dangerous situations that should be reported to the provider immediately.

M View Video: Danger Signs of Pregnancy

- Gush of fluid from the vagina (rupture of amniotic fluid) prior to 37 weeks of gestation
- Vaginal bleeding (placental problems such as abruption or previa)
- Abdominal pain (premature labor, abruptio placentae, or ectopic pregnancy)
- Changes in fetal activity (decreased fetal movement can indicate fetal distress)
- Persistent vomiting (hyperemesis gravidarum)
- Severe headaches (gestational hypertension)
- Elevated temperature (infection)
- Dysuria (urinary tract infection)
- Blurred vision (gestational hypertension)
- Edema of face and hands (gestational hypertension)
- Epigastric pain (gestational hypertension)
- Concurrent occurrence of flushed dry skin, fruity breath, rapid breathing, increased thirst and urination, and headache (hyperglycemia)
- Concurrent occurrence of clammy pale skin, weakness, tremors, irritability, and lightheadedness (hypoglycemia)

APPLICATION EXERCISES

1. A nurse is reinforcing teaching with a group of women who are pregnant about measures to relieve backache during pregnancy. The nurse should instruct the women on which of the following? (Select all that apply.)

_____ A. Avoid any lifting.

_____ B. Perform Kegel exercises twice a day.

_____ C. Perform the pelvic rock exercise every day.

_____ D. Use proper body mechanics.

_____ E. Avoid constrictive clothing.

2. A client who is at 8 weeks of gestation tells the nurse that she isn't sure she is happy about being pregnant. Which of the following is an appropriate response by the nurse to the client's statement?

A. "I will inform the provider that you are having these feelings."

B. "It is normal to have these feelings during the first few months of pregnancy."

C. "You should be happy that you are going to bring new life into the world."

D. "I am going to make an appointment with the counselor for you to discuss these thoughts."

3. A nurse is caring for a client who is pregnant and reviewing signs of complications the client should promptly report to the provider. Which of the following complications should the nurse include?

A. Vaginal bleeding

B. Swelling of the ankles

C. Heartburn after eating

D. Lightheadedness when lying on the back

4. A client who is at 7 weeks of gestation is experiencing nausea and vomiting in the morning. The nurse in the prenatal clinic reinforces teaching that should include which of the following instructions?

A. Eat crackers or plain toast before getting out of bed.

B. Awaken during the night to eat a snack.

C. Skip breakfast, and eat lunch after nausea has subsided.

D. Eat a large evening meal.

5. A nurse is reinforcing teaching with a group of clients who are pregnant about behaviors to avoid during pregnancy. Which of the following statements by a client indicates a need for further instruction?

    A. "I can have a glass of wine with dinner."

    B. "Smoking is a cause of low birth weight in babies."

    C. "Signs of infection should be reported to my doctor."

    D. "I should not take over-the-counter medications without checking with my obstetrician."

6. A nurse is caring for a client at 14 weeks of gestation and is reviewing self-care concepts regarding the prevention of urinary tract infections (UTIs). Which of the following should be included in the instruction? Use the ATI Active Learning Template: Basic Concept to complete this item to include the following sections:

    A. Underlying Principles: Describe two.

    B. Nursing Interventions: Describe two actions that decrease the risk of UTIs as they relate to each of the following types of interventions – When, Why, and How?

APPLICATION EXERCISES KEY

1. A. INCORRECT: Lifting can be done by using the legs, rather than the back.

    B. INCORRECT: Kegel exercises are done to strengthen the perineal muscles and do not relieve backache.

    C. **CORRECT:** The pelvic rock or tilt exercise stretches the muscles of the lower back and helps relieve lower-back pain.

    D. **CORRECT:** The use of proper body mechanics prevents back injury due to the incorrect use of muscles when lifting.

    E. INCORRECT: Avoiding constrictive clothing helps prevent urinary tract infections, vaginal infections, varicosities, and edema of the lower extremities.

    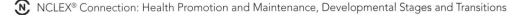 NCLEX® Connection: Health Promotion and Maintenance, Health Promotion/Disease Prevention

2. A. INCORRECT: This is a nontherapeutic response by the nurse and does not acknowledge the client's concerns.

    B. **CORRECT:** Feelings of ambivalence about pregnancy are normal during the first trimester.

    C. INCORRECT: This is a nontherapeutic response by the nurse and indicates disapproval.

    D. INCORRECT: This is a nontherapeutic response by the nurse and does not acknowledge the client's feelings.

    NCLEX® Connection: Health Promotion and Maintenance, Developmental Stages and Transitions

3. A. **CORRECT:** Vaginal bleeding indicates a potential complication of the placenta, such as placenta previa, and should be reported to the provider immediately.

    B. INCORRECT: Swelling of the ankles is a common occurrence during pregnancy and can be relieved by sitting with the legs elevated.

    C. INCORRECT: Heartburn occurs during pregnancy due to pressure on the stomach by the enlarging uterus. It can be relieved by eating small meals.

    D. INCORRECT: Supine hypotension can be experienced by the client who feels lightheaded or faint when lying on her back. The client should be instructed about the side-lying position to remove pressure of the uterus on the vena cava.

    NCLEX® Connection: Reduction of Risk Potential, Potential for Alterations in Body Systems

4. A. **CORRECT:** Nausea and vomiting during the first trimester can be relieved by eating crackers or plain toast 30 to 60 min prior to rising in the morning.

   B. INCORRECT: Eating during the night can cause heartburn and does not relieve nausea and vomiting during the first trimester.

   C. INCORRECT: Instruct the client to avoid an empty stomach for prolonged periods to reduce nausea and vomiting.

   D. INCORRECT: Eating a large meal in the evening can cause heartburn and does not relieve morning nausea and vomiting.

   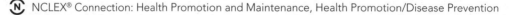 NCLEX® Connection: Health Promotion and Maintenance, Health Promotion/Disease Prevention

5. A. **CORRECT:** Alcohol should not be consumed during pregnancy due to the risk of birth defects.

   B. INCORRECT: Smoking during pregnancy results in low birth weight infants.

   C. INCORRECT: Signs of complications, such as infection, should be reported to the provider.

   D. INCORRECT: All medications should be reviewed with and approved by the provider.

   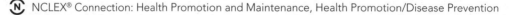 NCLEX® Connection: Health Promotion and Maintenance, High Risk Behaviors

6. *Using ATI Active Learning Template: Basic Concept*

   A. Underlying Principles
      - UTIs are common because of renal changes during pregnancy and the vaginal flora becoming more alkaline.

   B. Nursing Interventions
      - Decrease risk of UTIs by:
        - How, When: Wiping the perineal area from front to back after voiding.
        - How: Avoiding bubble baths.
        - How: Wearing cotton underpants. Avoiding tight-fitting pants.
        - How: Consuming at least 8 glasses of water per day.
        - How, Why: Urinating before and after intercourse to flush bacteria from the urethra that are present or introduced during intercourse.
        - How, Why: Urinating as soon as the urge occurs because retaining urine provides an environment for bacterial growth.
        - When, Why: Notifying her provider if her urine is foul-smelling, contains blood, or is cloudy so evaluation and early treatment can be initiated.

   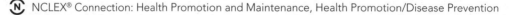 NCLEX® Connection: Health Promotion and Maintenance, Health Promotion/Disease Prevention

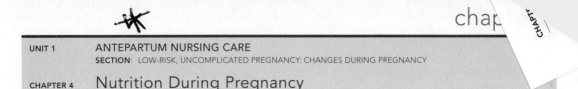
Overview

- Adequate nutritional intake during pregnancy is essential to promoting fetal and maternal health.

- Recommended weight gain during pregnancy is usually 11.5 to 16 kg (25 to 35 lb). The general rule is that clients should gain 1 to 2 kg (2.2 to 4.4 lb) during the first trimester and then approximately 0.4 kg (1 lb) per week for the last two trimesters. Underweight woman are advised to gain 28 to 40 lb; overweight women, 15 to 25 lb.

- It is important for the nurse to evaluate the pregnant client's nutritional choices, possible risk factors, and diet history. The nurse also should review specific nutritional guidelines for at-risk clients. Assistance is given to clients to develop a postpartum nutritional plan.

Data Collection and Interventions

- Obtain subjective and objective dietary information.
  - Journal of client's food habits, eating pattern, and cravings
  - Nutrition-related questionnaires
  - Client's weight on first prenatal visit and follow-up visits
  - Laboratory findings, such as Hgb and iron levels

Q
PCC • Determine client's caloric intake.
  - Have client record everything eaten. The nurse, dietitian, or client can identify the caloric value of each item. This record can provide better objective data about the client's nutrition status.

PLAN OF CARE FOR A PREGNANT CLIENT	
Expected Outcomes	› The client will consume the recommended dietary allowances/nutrients during her pregnancy.
Interventions	› The nurse reviews the client's dietary journal on the next prenatal visit.
	› The nurse provides educational materials regarding nutritional benefits to the mother and her newborn.
	› The nurse provides encouragement and answers questions that the client has regarding her dietary plans.
	› The nurse weighs the client and monitors for signs of inadequate weight gain.
	› The nurse makes a referral if needed.
Evaluation of the Plan	› Is there adequate weight gain?
	› Is the client compliant with the nursing plan of care?

- Instruct the client to adhere to and maintain the following during pregnancy.

  ○ An increase of 340 calories/day is recommended during the second trimester. An increase of 452 calories/day is recommended during the third trimester.

  ○ If the client is breastfeeding during the postpartum period, an additional intake of 330 calories/day is recommended during the first 6 months. An additional intake of 400 calories/day is recommended during the second 6 months.

  ○ Increasing protein intake is essential to basic growth. Also, the intake of foods high in folic acid is crucial for neurological development and the prevention of fetal neural tube defects. Foods high in folic acid include leafy vegetables, dried peas and beans, seeds, and orange juice. Breads, cereals, and other grains are fortified with folic acid. Increased intake of folic acid is encouraged for clients who wish to become pregnant and clients of childbearing age. It is recommended that 600 mcg of folic acid should be taken during pregnancy. Current recommendations for clients who are lactating include consuming 500 mcg of folic acid.

  ○ Iron supplements often are added to the prenatal plan to facilitate an increase of the maternal RBC mass. Iron is best absorbed between meals and when given with a source of vitamin C. Milk and caffeine interfere with the absorption of iron supplements. Food sources of iron include beef liver, red meats, fish, poultry, dried peas and beans, and fortified cereals and breads. A stool softener might need to be added to decrease constipation experienced with iron supplements.

  ○ Calcium, which is important to a developing fetus, is involved in bone and teeth formation.

    ▪ Sources of calcium include milk, calcium-fortified soy milk, fortified orange juice, nuts, legumes, and dark green leafy vegetables. Daily recommendation is 1,000 mg/day for pregnant and nonpregnant women over the age of 19, and 1,300 mg/day for those under 19 years of age.

  ○ 2 to 3 L of fluids is recommended daily. Preferred fluids are water, fruit juice, and milk.

  ○ Caffeine intake should be limited to 200 mg/day. The equivalent of 360 mL/day of coffee can increase the risk of a spontaneous abortion or fetal intrauterine growth restriction.

  ○ It is recommended that women abstain from alcohol consumption during pregnancy.

Risk Factors to Ensuring Adequate Nutrition During Pregnancy

- Age, culture, education, and socioeconomic issues can affect adequate nutrition during pregnancy. Also, certain conditions specific to each client can inhibit adequate caloric intake.

  ○ Adolescents can have poor nutritional habits (a diet low in vitamins and protein, not taking prescribed iron supplements).

  ○ Vegetarians can have low protein, calcium, iron, zinc, and vitamin B_{12}.

  ○ Nausea and vomiting during pregnancy.

  ○ Anemia.

  ○ Eating disorders, such as anorexia nervosa or bulimia nervosa.

- Pregnant clients diagnosed with the appetite disorder pica (craving to eat nonfood substances such as dirt or red clay). This disorder can diminish the amount of nutritional foods ingested.

- Excessive weight gain can lead to macrosomia and labor complications.

- Inability to gain weight can result in low birth weight of the newborn.

- Financially unable to purchase/access food. Therefore, the nurse should advise the client about the Women, Infants and Children (WIC) programs, which are federally funded state programs for pregnant women and their children (up to 5 years old).

Dietary Complications During Pregnancy

- Nausea and constipation are common during pregnancy.

  - For nausea, tell the client to eat dry crackers or toast, and avoid alcohol, caffeine, fats, and spices. Also avoid drinking fluids with meals, and DO NOT take a medication to control nausea without first checking with the provider.

  - For constipation, increase fluid consumption and include extra fiber in the diet. Fruits, vegetables, and whole grains all contain fiber.

- Maternal phenylketonuria (PKU) is a maternal genetic disease in which high levels of phenylalanine pose a danger to the fetus.

  - It is important for the client to resume the PKU diet for at least 3 months prior to pregnancy and continue the diet throughout pregnancy.

  - The diet includes foods that are low in phenylalanine. Foods high in protein, such as fish, poultry, meat, eggs, nuts, and dairy products, must be avoided due to high phenylalanine levels.

  - The client's blood phenylalanine levels are monitored during pregnancy.

  - These interventions can prevent fetal complications, such as mental retardation and behavioral problems.

Creating a Postpartum Nutritional Plan

- A lactating woman's nutritional plan includes the following instructions.

  - Increase protein and calorie intake while adhering to a recommended, well-balanced diet.

  - Increase oral fluids, but avoid alcohol and caffeine.

  - Avoid food substances that do not agree with the newborn (foods that can cause altered bowel function).

  - The client should take calcium supplements if she consumes an inadequate amount of dietary calcium.

- A nutritional plan for a woman who is not breastfeeding should include resumption of a previously recommended well-balanced diet.

APPLICATION EXERCISES

1. A nurse in a prenatal clinic is providing instructions to a client who is in the 8th week of gestation. The client states that she does not like milk. What is a good source of calcium that the nurse can recommend to the client?

    A. Dark green, leafy vegetables

    B. Deep red or orange vegetables

    C. White breads and rice

    D. Meat, poultry, and fish

2. A nurse in a prenatal clinic is caring for a group of clients. Which of the following clients should the nurse be concerned about regarding weight gain?

    A. 1.8 kg (4 lb) weight gain and is in her first trimester

    B. 3.6 kg (7.9 lb) weight gain and is in her first trimester

    C. 6.8 kg (15 lb) weight gain and is in her second trimester

    D. 11.3 kg (24.9 lb) weight gain and is in her third trimester

3. A nurse in a clinic is reinforcing teaching with a client of childbearing age about recommended folic acid supplements. Which of the following defects can occur in the fetus or neonate as a result of folic acid deficiency?

    A. Iron deficiency anemia

    B. Poor bone formation

    C. Macrosomic fetus

    D. Neural tube defects

4. A nurse is reviewing a new prescription for iron supplements with a client who is in the 8th week of gestation and has iron deficiency anemia. The nurse should advise the client to take the iron supplements with which of the following?

    A. Ice water

    B. Low-fat or whole milk

    C. Tea or coffee

    D. Orange juice

5. A nurse is reviewing postpartum nutrition needs with a group of new mothers who are breastfeeding their newborns. Which of the following statements by a member of the group requires clarification?

   A. "I am glad I can have my morning coffee."

   B. "I know that certain foods that I eat will affect my baby."

   C. "I will continue adding 330 calories per day to my diet."

   D. "I will continue my calcium supplements because I don't like milk."

6. A nurse manager in a prenatal clinic is preparing an in-service education program for a group of newly licensed nurses about risk factors to ensuring adequate nutrition during pregnancy. Which of the following should be included in this presentation? Use the ATI Active Learning Template: Basic Concept to answer this item and include the following:

   A. Underlying Principles:
      - Identify one that is age-related.
      - Identify two that are related to culture/lifestyle.
      - Identify one that is related to a socioeconomic factor.
      - Identify two that are related to dietary complications during pregnancy.

   B. Nursing Intervention: Describe a federal program that is available to woman and children to provide nutrition support.

APPLICATION EXERCISES KEY

1. A. **CORRECT:** Good sources of calcium for bone and teeth formation include low-oxalate, dark-green, leafy vegetables, such as kale, artichokes, and turnip greens.

    B. INCORRECT: Deep red or orange vegetables are good sources of vitamins C and A.

    C. INCORRECT: White breads and rice do not contain high levels of calcium.

    D. INCORRECT: Meat, poultry, and fish are sources of protein but do not contain high levels of calcium.

     NCLEX® Connection: Basic Care and Comfort, Nutrition and Oral Hydration

2. A. INCORRECT: This client has gained the appropriate weight of 3 to 4 lb for a client in the first trimester.

    B. **CORRECT:** The nurse should be concerned about this client because she has exceeded the expected 3- to 4-lb weight gain of a client in the first trimester.

    C. INCORRECT: This client has gained the appropriate weight of 3 to 4 lb in the first trimester and approximately 1 lb/week in the second trimester.

    D. INCORRECT: This client is within the recommended weight gain of 25 to 35 lb during the third trimester.

     NCLEX® Connection: Reduction of Risk Potential, Potential for Alterations in Body Systems

3. A. INCORRECT: Iron deficiency anemia is the result of a lack of iron-rich dietary sources, such as meat, chicken, and fish.

    B. INCORRECT: Calcium deficiency can result in poor bone and teeth formation.

    C. INCORRECT: Maternal obesity can lead to a macrosomic fetus.

    D. **CORRECT:** Neural tube defects are caused by folic acid deficiency. Food sources of folic acid include fresh green, leafy vegetables, liver, peanuts, cereals, and whole-grain breads.

     NCLEX® Connection: Health Promotion and Maintenance, Health Promotion/Disease Prevention

4. A. INCORRECT: Water does not promote absorption of iron, but drinking plenty of water can prevent constipation, which is an adverse effect of iron supplements.

    B. INCORRECT: Milk interferes with iron absorption.

    C. INCORRECT: Caffeine, found in tea and coffee, can interfere with iron absorption. It also should be limited to 200 mg/day because it increases the risk of spontaneous abortion and fetal intrauterine growth restriction.

    D. **CORRECT:** Orange juice contains vitamin C, which aids in the absorption of iron.

    Ⓝ NCLEX® Connection: Pharmacological Therapies, Expected Actions/Outcomes

5. A. **CORRECT:** Women who are breastfeeding should avoid caffeine intake because it affects iron absorption and infant weight gain.

    B. INCORRECT: Foods ingested by the mother, especially gas-producing foods, can affect breast milk and the breastfeeding infant.

    C. INCORRECT: Women who are breastfeeding require an additional 330 calories/day to support adequate nutrition during the first 6 months of lactation.

    D. INCORRECT: Postpartum women who are at risk for inadequate dietary calcium should continue taking calcium supplements during lactation.

    Ⓝ NCLEX® Connection: Health Promotion and Maintenance, Health Promotion/Disease Prevention

6. *Using the ATI Active Learning Template: Basic Concept*

    A. Underlying Principles

        • Age-related: Adolescents an have poor nutritional habits during pregnancy.

        • Culture/lifestyle: Vegetarians can have diets low in protein, calcium, zinc, and vitamin B_{12}. Excessive weight gain can lead to macrosomia and labor complications.

        • Socioeconomic factor: Inability to purchase or access foods can limit nutrition during pregnancy.

        • Dietary complications: Nausea and vomiting during pregnancy, anemia, eating disorders (anorexia nervosa or bulimia nervosa), inability to gain weight, (an appetite disorder).

    B. Nursing Intervention

        • Women, Infants and Children (WIC) is a federally funded state program that provides nutritional support to pregnant women and their children (up to 5 years old).

    Ⓝ NCLEX® Connection: Basic Care and Comfort, Nutrition and Oral Hydration

chapter 5

Overview

- This chapter includes the diagnostic tests that determine the well-being of a fetus during pregnancy.

- The diagnostic procedures to be reviewed include ultrasound (abdominal, transvaginal, Doppler), biophysical profile, nonstress test, contraction stress test (nipple, oxytocin [Pitocin]), and amniocentesis. Additional diagnostic procedures for high-risk pregnancy include percutaneous umbilical cord blood sampling, chorionic villus sampling, quad marker screening, and maternal serum alpha-fetoprotein.

DIAGNOSTIC PROCEDURE AND NURSING MANAGEMENT: ULTRASOUND (ABDOMINAL, TRANSVAGINAL, DOPPLER)

Overview

- Ultrasound – a procedure lasting approximately 20 min that consists of high-frequency sound waves used to visualize internal organs and tissues by producing a real-time, three-dimensional image of the developing fetus and maternal structures (FHR, pelvic anatomy). An ultrasound allows for early diagnosis of complications, permits earlier interventions, and thereby decreases neonatal and maternal morbidity and mortality. There are three types of ultrasound: external abdominal, transvaginal, and Doppler.

  ○ External abdominal ultrasound – a safe, noninvasive, painless procedure whereby an ultrasound transducer is moved over a client's abdomen to obtain an image. An abdominal ultrasound is more useful after the first trimester when the gravid uterus is larger.

  ○ Internal transvaginal ultrasound – an invasive procedure in which a probe is inserted vaginally to allow for a more accurate evaluation. An advantage of this procedure is that it does not require a full bladder.

    ■ It is especially useful in clients who are obese and those in the first trimester to detect an ectopic pregnancy, identify abnormalities, and establish gestational age.

    ■ A transvaginal ultrasound also can be used in the third trimester in conjunction with abdominal scanning to evaluate for preterm labor.

  ○ Doppler ultrasound blood flow analysis – a noninvasive external ultrasound method to study the maternal-fetal blood flow by measuring the velocity at which RBCs travel in the uterine and fetal vessels using a handheld ultrasound device that reflects sound waves from a moving target. It is especially useful in fetal intrauterine growth restriction (IUGR) and poor placental perfusion, and as an adjunct in pregnancies at risk because of hypertension, diabetes mellitus, multiple fetuses, or preterm labor.

- Indications for the use of an ultrasound during pregnancy

  ○ Potential diagnoses

    ■ Confirming pregnancy

    ■ Confirming gestational age by biparietal diameter (side-to-side) measurement

    ■ Identifying multifetal pregnancy

- Site of fetal implantation (uterine or ectopic)
- Assessing fetal growth and development
- Assessing maternal structures
- Confirming fetal viability or death
- Ruling out or verifying fetal abnormalities
- Locating the site of placental attachment
- Determining amniotic fluid volume
- Fetal movement observation (fetal heartbeat, breathing, and activity)
- Placental grading (evaluating placental maturation)
- Adjunct for other procedures (e.g., amniocentesis, biophysical profile)
  - Client presentation
    - Vaginal bleeding evaluation
    - Questionable fundal height measurement in relationship to gestational weeks
    - Reports of decreased fetal movements
    - Preterm labor
    - Questionable rupture of membranes
- Nursing actions for an ultrasound
  - Preparation of client
    - Explain the procedure to the client and that it presents no known risk to her or her fetus.
    - Advise the client to drink 1 to 2 quarts of fluid prior to the ultrasound to fill the bladder, lift and stabilize the uterus, displace the bowel, and act as an echolucent to better reflect sound waves to obtain a better image of the fetus.
    - Assist the client into a supine position with a wedge placed under her right hip to displace the uterus (prevents supine hypotension).
  - Ongoing care
    - Apply an ultrasonic/transducer gel to the client's abdomen before the transducer is moved over the skin to obtain a better fetal image, ensuring that the gel is at room temperature or warmer.
    - Allow the client to empty her bladder at the termination of the procedure.
- Nursing actions for a transvaginal ultrasound
  - Preparation of client
    - Assist the client into a lithotomy position. The vaginal probe is covered with a protective device, lubricated with a water-soluble gel, and the client or examiner inserts the probe.
  - Ongoing care
    - During the procedure, the position of the probe or tilt of the table can be changed to facilitate the complete view of the pelvis.
    - Inform the client that pressure can be felt as the probe is moved.
- Client education
  - Fetal and maternal structures can be pointed out to the client as the ultrasound procedure is performed.

DIAGNOSTIC PROCEDURE AND NURSING MANAGEMENT:
BIOPHYSICAL PROFILE

Overview

- Biophysical profile (BPP) – uses a real-time ultrasound to visualize physical and physiological characteristics of the fetus and observe for fetal biophysical responses to stimuli.

- BPP assesses fetal well-being by measuring the following five variables with a score of 2 for each normal finding, and 0 for each abnormal finding for each variable.

  - Reactive FHR (reactive nonstress test) = 2; nonreactive = 0.

  - Fetal breathing movements (at least 1 episode of greater than 30 seconds duration in 30 min) = 2; absent or less than 30 seconds duration = 0.

  - Gross body movements (at least 3 body or limb extensions with return to flexion in 30 min) = 2; less than three episodes = 0.

  - Fetal tone (at least 1 episode of extension with return to flexion) = 2; slow extension and flexion, lack of flexion, or absent movement = 0.

  - Qualitative amniotic fluid volume (at least one pocket of fluid that measures at least 2 cm in two perpendicular planes) = 2; pockets absent or less than 2 cm = 0.

- Interpretation of findings

  - Total score of 8 to 10 is normal; low risk of chronic fetal asphyxia

  - 4 to 6 is abnormal; suspect chronic fetal asphyxia

  - Less than 4 is abnormal; strongly suspect chronic fetal asphyxia

- Potential diagnoses

  - Nonreactive stress test

  - Suspected oligohydramnios or polyhydramnios

  - Suspected fetal hypoxemia and/or hypoxia

- Client presentation

  - Premature rupture of membranes

  - Maternal infection

  - Decreased fetal movement

  - Intrauterine growth restriction

- Nursing Actions

  - Prepare the client following the same nursing management principles as those used for an ultrasound.

DIAGNOSTIC PROCEDURE AND NURSING MANAGEMENT:
NONSTRESS TEST (NST)

Overview

- Nonstress test (NST) – most widely used technique for antepartum evaluation of fetal well-being performed during the third trimester. It is a noninvasive procedure that monitors response of the FHR to fetal movement. A Doppler transducer (used to monitor the FHR) and a tocotransducer (used to monitor uterine contractions) are attached externally to a client's abdomen to obtain tracing strips. The client pushes a button attached to the monitor whenever she feels a fetal movement, which is then noted on the tracing. This allows a nurse to monitor the FHR in relationship to the fetal movement.

- Indications for the use of an NST during pregnancy
  - ○ Potential diagnoses
    - ▪ Monitoring for an intact fetal CNS during the third trimester.
    - ▪ Ruling out the risk for fetal death in clients who have diabetes mellitus. Used twice a week or until after 28 weeks of gestation.
  - ○ Client presentation
    - ▪ Decreased fetal movement
    - ▪ Intrauterine growth restriction
    - ▪ Postmaturity
    - ▪ Gestational diabetes mellitus
    - ▪ Gestational hypertension
    - ▪ Maternal chronic hypertension
    - ▪ History of previous fetal demise
    - ▪ Advanced maternal age
    - ▪ Sickle cell disease
    - ▪ Isoimmunization

- Interpretation of findings
  - ○ The NST is interpreted as reactive if the FHR is a normal baseline rate with moderate variability, accelerates to 15 beats/min for at least 15 seconds, and occurs two or more times during a 20-min period.

 View Image: Reactive NST

- ○ Nonreactive NST indicates that the fetal heart rate does not accelerate adequately with fetal movement. It does not meet the above criteria after 40 min. Additional assessment, such as a contraction stress test (CST) or biophysical profile (BPP), is indicated.

- Nursing actions
  - ○ Preparation of client
    - ▪ Seat the client in a reclining chair, or place in a semi-Fowler's or left-lateral position.
    - ▪ Apply conduction gel to the client's abdomen.
    - ▪ Apply two belts to the client's abdomen, and attach the FHR and uterine contraction monitors.

- Ongoing care
  - Instruct the client to press the button on the handheld event marker each time she feels the fetus move.
  - If there are no fetal movements (fetus sleeping), vibroacoustic stimulation (sound source, usually laryngeal stimulator) can be activated for 3 seconds on the maternal abdomen over the fetal head to awaken a sleeping fetus.
- Miscellaneous
  - Disadvantages of a NST include a high rate of false nonreactive results with the fetal movement response blunted by sleep cycles of the fetus, fetal immaturity, maternal medications, and chronic smoking.

DIAGNOSTIC PROCEDURE AND NURSING MANAGEMENT: CONTRACTION STRESS TEST (CST)

Overview

- Nipple stimulated CST consists of a woman lightly brushing her palm across her nipple for 2 min, which causes the pituitary gland to release endogenous oxytocin, and then stopping the nipple stimulation when a contraction begins. The same process is repeated after a 5-min rest period.
  - Analysis of the FHR response to contractions (which decrease placental blood flow) determines how the fetus will tolerate the stress of labor. A pattern of at least three contractions within a 10-min time period with duration of 40 to 60 seconds each must be obtained to use for assessment data.
  - Hyperstimulation of the uterus (uterine contraction longer than 90 seconds or more frequent than every 2 min) should be avoided by stimulating the nipple intermittently with rest periods in between and avoiding bimanual stimulation of both nipples unless stimulation of one nipple is unsuccessful.
- Oxytocin (Pitocin) administration CST is used if nipple stimulation fails and consists of the IV administration of oxytocin to induce uterine contractions.
  - Contractions started with oxytocin can be difficult to stop and can lead to preterm labor.
- Indications for the use of a contraction stress test during pregnancy
  - Potential diagnoses
    - High-risk pregnancies (gestational diabetes mellitus, postterm pregnancy)
    - Nonreactive stress test
  - Client presentation
    - Decreased fetal movement
    - Intrauterine growth restriction
    - Postmaturity
    - Gestational diabetes mellitus
    - Gestational hypertension

- Maternal chronic hypertension
- History of previous fetal demise
- Advanced maternal age
- Sickle-cell disease

- Interpretation of findings
  - A negative CST (normal finding) is indicated if within a 10-min period, with three uterine contractions, there are no late decelerations of the FHR.
  - A positive CST (abnormal finding) is indicated with persistent and consistent late decelerations on more than half of the contractions. This is suggestive of uteroplacental insufficiency. Variable deceleration may indicate cord compression, and early decelerations can indicate fetal head compression. Based on these findings, the provider might determine to induce labor or perform a cesarean birth.

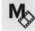 View Image: Positive CST

- Nursing Actions
  - Preparation of client
    - Obtain a baseline of the FHR, fetal movement, and contractions for 10 to 20 min, and document.
    - Explain the procedure to the client, and obtain informed consent.
    - Complete data collection without artificial stimulation if contractions are occurring spontaneously.
  - Ongoing care
    - Initiate nipple stimulation if there are no contractions. Instruct the client to roll a nipple between her thumb and fingers or brush her palm across her nipple. The client should stop when a uterine contraction begins.
    - Monitor and provide adequate rest periods for the client to avoid hyperstimulation of the uterus.
  - Interventions
    - The client should receive IV oxytocin administration if nipple stimulation fails to elicit a sufficient uterine contraction pattern. If hyperstimulation of the uterus and/or preterm labor occurs, do the following.
      - Monitor for contractions lasting longer than 90 seconds and/or occurring more frequently than every 2 min.
      - Monitor the administration of tocolytics as prescribed.
      - Maintain bed rest during the procedure.
      - Observe the client for 30 min afterward to see that contractions have ceased and preterm labor does not begin.
- Complications
  - Potential for preterm labor

DIAGNOSTIC PROCEDURE AND NURSING MANAGEMENT: AMNIOCENTESIS

Overview

- Amniocentesis – the aspiration of amniotic fluid for analysis by insertion of a needle transabdominally into a client's uterus and amniotic sac under direct ultrasound guidance locating the placenta and determining the position of the fetus. It can be performed after 14 weeks of gestation.

- Indications for the use of an amniocentesis during pregnancy
  - Potential diagnoses
    - Previous birth with a chromosomal anomaly
    - A parent who is a carrier of a chromosomal anomaly
    - Family history of neural tube defects
    - Prenatal diagnosis of a genetic disorder or congenital anomaly of the fetus
    - Alpha-fetoprotein level for fetal abnormalities
    - Lung maturity assessment
    - Fetal hemolytic disease
    - Meconium in the amniotic fluid

- Interpretation of findings
  - Alpha-fetoprotein (AFP) can be measured from the amniotic fluid between 16 and 18 weeks of gestation and can be used to assess for neural tube defects in the fetus or chromosomal disorders. Can be evaluated to follow up a high level of AFP in maternal serum.
    - High levels of AFP are associated with neural tube defects, such as anencephaly (incomplete development of fetal skull and brain), spina bifida (open spine), or omphalocele (abdominal wall defect). High AFP levels also can be present with normal multifetal pregnancies.
    - Low levels of AFP are associated with chromosomal disorders (Down syndrome) or gestational trophoblastic disease (hydatidiform mole).
  - Tests for fetal lung maturity can be performed if gestation is less than 37 weeks, in the event of a rupture of membranes, for preterm labor, or for a complication indicating a cesarean birth. Amniotic fluid is tested to determine whether the fetal lungs are mature enough to adapt to extrauterine life, or if the fetus likely will have respiratory distress. Determination is made whether the fetus should be removed immediately or if the fetus requires more time in utero with the administration of glucocorticoids to promote fetal lung maturity.
    - Fetal lung tests
      - Lecithin/sphingomyelin (L/S) ratio – a 2:1 ratio indicating fetal lung maturity (2.5:1 or 3:1 for a client who has diabetes mellitus).
      - Presence of phosphatidylglycerol (PG) – absence of PG is associated with respiratory distress

- Preprocedure for an amniocentesis
  - Nursing actions
    - Explain the procedure to the client, and obtain informed consent.
  - Client education
    - Instruct the client to empty her bladder prior to the procedure to reduce its size and reduce the risk of inadvertent puncture.

- Intraprocedure
  - Nursing actions
    - Obtain client's baseline vital signs and FHR, and document prior to the procedure.
    - Assist client into a supine position, and place a wedge under her right hip to displace the uterus off the vena cava, and place a drape over the client exposing only her abdomen.
    - Prepare client for an ultrasound to locate the placenta.
    - Cleanse client's abdomen with an antiseptic solution prior to the administration of a local anesthetic by the provider.
  - Client education
    - Advise the client that she will feel slight pressure as the needle is inserted. She should continue breathing because holding her breath will lower the diaphragm against the uterus and shift the intrauterine contents.
- Postprocedure
  - Nursing actions
    - Monitor the client's vital signs, FHR, and uterine contractions throughout and 30 min following the procedure.
    - Have the client rest for 30 min.
    - The client should receive $Rh_o(D)$ immune globulin (RhoGAM) to the client if she is Rh-negative (standard practice after an amniocentesis for all women who are Rh-negative to protect against Rh isoimmunization).
  - Client education
    - Advise the client to report to the provider if she experiences fever, chills, leakage of fluid, or bleeding from the insertion site, decreased fetal movement, vaginal bleeding, or uterine contractions after the procedure.
    - Encourage the client to drink plenty of liquids and rest for 24 hr postprocedure.
  - Complications
    - Amniotic fluid emboli
    - Maternal or fetal hemorrhage
    - Fetomaternal hemorrhage with Rh isoimmunization
    - Maternal or fetal infection
    - Inadvertent fetal damage or anomalies involving limbs
    - Fetal death
    - Inadvertent maternal intestinal or bladder damage
    - Spontaneous abortion or preterm labor
    - Premature rupture of membranes
    - Leakage of amniotic fluid
  - Nursing actions
    - Monitor the client's vital signs, temperature, respiratory status, FHR, uterine contractions, and vaginal discharge for amniotic fluid or bleeding.
    - Administer medication as prescribed.
    - Offer support and reassurance.

DIAGNOSTIC PROCEDURE AND NURSING MANAGEMENT (HIGH-RISK PREGNANCY): PERCUTANEOUS UMBILICAL BLOOD SAMPLING

Overview

- Percutaneous umbilical blood sampling (PUBS) – the most common method used for fetal blood sampling and transfusion. This procedure obtains fetal blood from the umbilical cord by passing a fine-gauge, fiber-optic scope (fetoscope) into the amniotic sac using the amniocentesis technique. The needle is advanced into the umbilical cord under ultrasound guidance, and blood is aspirated from the umbilical vein. Blood studies from the cordocentesis may consist of:
  - Kleihauer-Betke test that ensures that fetal blood was obtained.
  - CBC count with differential.
  - Indirect Coombs test for Rh antibodies.
  - Karyotyping (visualization of chromosomes).
  - Blood gases.
- Indications for the use of PUBS
  - Potential diagnoses
    - Fetal blood type, RBC, and chromosomal disorders
    - Karyotyping of malformed fetuses
    - Fetal infection
    - Altered acid-base balance of fetuses with IUGR
- Interpretation of findings
  - Evaluates for isoimmune fetal hemolytic anemia and assesses the need for a fetal blood transfusion.
- Nursing actions
  - Administer medication as prescribed.
  - Offer support.
- Complications
  - Cord laceration
  - Preterm labor
  - Amnionitis
  - Hematoma
  - Fetomaternal hemorrhage

DIAGNOSTIC PROCEDURE AND NURSING MANAGEMENT (HIGH-RISK PREGNANCY): CHORIONIC VILLUS SAMPLING

Overview

- Chorionic villus sampling (CVS) – assessment of a portion of the developing placenta (chorionic villi), which is aspirated through a thin sterile catheter or syringe inserted through the abdominal wall or intravaginally through the cervix under ultrasound guidance and analyzed.
  - CVS is a first-trimester alternative to amniocentesis, with one of its advantages being an earlier diagnosis of any abnormalities. CVS can be performed between 10 and 13 weeks of gestation, and rapid results with chromosome studies are available in 24 to 48 hr following aspiration.
- Indications for the use of CVS during pregnancy
  - Potential diagnoses
    - Women at risk for giving birth to a neonate who has a genetic chromosomal abnormality (cannot determine spina bifida or anencephaly)
  - Client education
    - Instruct the client to drink plenty of fluid to fill the bladder prior to the procedure to assist in positioning the uterus for catheter insertion.
    - Provide ongoing education and support.
- Complications
  - Spontaneous abortion (higher risk with CVS than with amniocentesis)
  - Risk for fetal limb loss
  - Chorioamnionitis and rupture of membranes
- Miscellaneous
  - The advantage of an earlier diagnosis should be weighed against the increased risk of fetal anomalies and death.

DIAGNOSTIC PROCEDURE AND NURSING MANAGEMENT (HIGH-RISK PREGNANCY): QUAD MARKER AND ALPHA-FETOPROTEIN (AFP) SCREENING

Overview

- Description of procedure
  - Quad marker screening – a blood test that ascertains information about the likelihood of fetal birth defects. It does not diagnose the actual defect. It can be performed instead of the maternal serum alpha-fetoprotein (MSAFP), yielding more reliable findings. Includes testing for:
    - Human chorionic gonadotropin (hCG) – a hormone produced by the placenta
    - Alpha-fetoprotein (AFP) – a protein produced by the fetus
    - Estriol – a protein produced by the fetus and placenta
    - Inhibin-A – a protein produced by the ovaries and placenta
- Indications
  - Client presentation
    - Preferred at 16 to 18 weeks of gestation
    - Women at risk for giving birth to a neonate who has a genetic chromosomal abnormality
- Interpretation of findings
  - Low levels of AFP can indicate a risk for Down syndrome.
  - High levels of AFP can indicate a risk for neural tube defects.
  - Higher levels than the expected reference range of hCG and inhibin-A indicates a risk for Down syndrome.
  - Lower levels than the expected reference range of estriol can indicate a risk for Down syndrome.
- Description of procedure
  - MSAFP is a screening tool used to detect neural tube defects. Clients who have abnormal findings should be referred for a quad marker screening, genetic counseling, ultrasound, and an amniocentesis.
- Indications
  - Potential diagnoses
    - All pregnant clients, preferably between 16 to 18 weeks of gestation
- Interpretation of findings
  - High levels can indicate a neural tube defect or open abdominal defect.
  - Lower levels can indicate Down syndrome.
- Nursing Actions
  - Preparation of a client
    - Discuss testing with the client.
    - Assist with the collection of a blood sample.
    - Offer support and education as needed.

APPLICATION EXERCISES

1. A nurse is caring for a client and reviewing the findings of the client's biophysical profile (BPP). Which of the following variables are included in this test? (Select all that apply.)

_____ A. Fetal weight

_____ B. Fetal breathing movement

_____ C. Fetal tone

_____ D. Reactive FHR

_____ E. Amniotic fluid volume

2. A nurse is caring for a client who is in preterm labor and is scheduled to undergo an amniocentesis to assess fetal lung maturity. Which of the following is a test for fetal lung maturity?

A. Alpha-fetoprotein (AFP)

B. Lecithin/sphingomyelin (L/S) ratio

C. Kleihauer-Betke test

D. Indirect Coombs test

3. A nurse is caring for a client who is pregnant and undergoing a nonstress test. The client asks why the nurse is using an acoustic vibration device. Which of the following is an appropriate response by the nurse?

A. "It is used to stimulate uterine contractions."

B. "It will decrease the incidence of uterine contractions."

C. "It lulls the fetus to sleep."

D. "It awakens a sleeping fetus."

4. A nurse is reinforcing teaching with a client who is pregnant about the amniocentesis procedure. Which of the following statements by the client requires clarification?

A. "I will report cramping or signs of infection to the physician."

B. "I should drink lots of fluids during the 24 hours following the procedure."

C. "I need to have a full bladder at the time of the procedure."

D. "The test is done to detect genetic abnormalities."

5. A nurse is caring for a client who is pregnant and is to undergo a contraction stress test (CST). Which of the following findings are indications for this procedure? (Select all that apply.)

_____ A. Decreased fetal movement

_____ B. Intrauterine growth restriction (IUGR)

_____ C. Postmaturity

_____ D. Advanced maternal age

_____ E. Amniotic fluid emboli

6. A nurse in a prenatal clinic is orienting a recently hired nurse about how to perform a nonstress test (NST). What should be included in the orientation? Use the ATI Active Learning Template: Diagnostic Procedure to complete this item to include the following:

A. Indications: Identify three that relate to the status of the fetus.

B. Interpretation of Findings: Describe a nonreactive NST.

C. Nursing Actions: Two preprocedure, one intraprocedure.

APPLICATION EXERCISES KEY

1. A. INCORRECT: Fetal weight is not one of the variables included in the BPP.

    B. **CORRECT:** Fetal breathing movements are a variable included in the BPP.

    C. **CORRECT:** Fetal tone is a variable included in the BPP.

    D. **CORRECT:** Reactive FHR is a variable included in the BPP.

    E. **CORRECT:** Amniotic fluid volume is a variable included in the BPP.

    Ⓝ NCLEX® Connection: Reduction of Risk Potential, Laboratory Values

2. A. INCORRECT: AFP is a test to assess for fetal neural tube defects or chromosome disorders.

    B. **CORRECT:** A test of the L/S ratio is done as a part of an amniocentesis to determine fetal lung maturity.

    C. INCORRECT: A Kleihauer-Betke test is used to verify that fetal blood is present during a percutaneous umbilical blood sampling procedure.

    D. INCORRECT: An indirect Coombs test detects Rh antibodies in the mother's blood.

    Ⓝ NCLEX® Connection: Reduction of Risk Potential, Diagnostic Tests

3. A. INCORRECT: The acoustic vibration device does not stimulate the uterus.

    B. INCORRECT: The acoustic vibration device has no effect on the uterine muscles.

    C. INCORRECT: The acoustic vibration device stimulates a sleeping fetus.

    D. **CORRECT:** The acoustic vibration device is activated for 3 seconds on the maternal abdomen over the fetal head to awaken a sleeping fetus.

    Ⓝ NCLEX® Connection: Health Promotion and Maintenance, Ante/Intra/Postpartum and Newborn Care

4.   A. INCORRECT: Cramping and signs of infection following the procedure should be reported to the provider.

   B. INCORRECT: The client is encouraged to drink extra fluids and rest during the 24 hr following an amniocentesis.

   C. **CORRECT:** The client's bladder should be empty to avoid an inadvertent puncture during the procedure.

   D. INCORRECT: Amniotic fluid is tested to identify fetal genetic defects.

   Ⓝ NCLEX® Connection: Reduction of Risk Potential, Diagnostic Tests

5.   A. **CORRECT:** Decreased fetal movement is an indication for a CST.

   B. **CORRECT:** IUGR is an indication for a CST.

   C. **CORRECT:** Postmaturity is an indication for a CST.

   D. **CORRECT:** Advanced maternal age is an indication for a CST.

   E. INCORRECT: Amniotic fluid emboli are a complication of an amniocentesis.

   Ⓝ NCLEX® Connection: Reduction of Risk Potential, Diagnostic Tests

6.   *Using the ATI Active Learning Template: Diagnostic Procedure*

   A. Indications

   - Assessment for intact fetal CNS during the third trimester
   - Rule out fetal death in a client who has diabetes mellitus
   - Decreased fetal movement
   - Intrauterine growth restriction
   - Postmaturity

   B. Interpretation of Findings

   - Nonreactive NST: Fetal heart rate does not accelerate by 15 beats/min above the baseline FHR for at least 15 seconds at least two or more times during a period of 20 min.

   C. Nursing Actions

   - Preprocedure
      ○ Seat the client in a reclining chair in a semi-Fowler's or left-lateral position.
      ○ Apply conduction gel to the client's abdomen.
      ○ Apply the Doppler transducer and the tocotransducer.
   - Intraprocedure
      ○ Instruct the client to depress the event marker button each time she feels fetal movement.

   Ⓝ NCLEX® Connection: Health Promotion and Maintenance, Ante/Intra/Postpartum and Newborn Care

chapter 6

Overview

- Vaginal bleeding during pregnancy is always abnormal and must be investigated to determine the cause. It can impair both the outcome of the pregnancy and the mother's life.

- The primary causes of bleeding are summarized in the following table according to common causes during each trimester of pregnancy.

SUMMARY OF CAUSES OF BLEEDING DURING PREGNANCY		
Time	Complication	Signs and symptoms
› First trimester	› Spontaneous abortion	› Vaginal bleeding, uterine cramping, and partial or complete expulsion of products of conception
	› Ectopic pregnancy	› Abrupt unilateral lower-quadrant abdominal pain with or without vaginal bleeding
› Second trimester	› Gestational trophoblastic disease	› Uterine size increasing abnormally fast, abnormally high levels of hCG, nausea and increased emesis, no fetus present on ultrasound, and scant or profuse dark brown or red vaginal bleeding
› Third trimester	› Placenta previa	› Painless vaginal bleeding
	› Abruptio placenta	› Vaginal bleeding, sharp abdominal pain, and tender rigid uterus

- Other Causes of Bleeding
  - Recurrent premature dilation of the cervix
    - Painless bleeding with cervical dilation leading to fetal expulsion
  - Preterm labor
    - Pink-stained vaginal discharge, uterine contractions becoming regular, cervical dilation and effacement

---

SPONTANEOUS ABORTION

Overview

- Spontaneous abortion is when a pregnancy is terminated before 20 weeks of gestation (the point of fetal viability) or a fetal weight less than 500 g.

- Types of abortion are clinically classified according to clinical manifestations and whether the products of conception are partially or completely retained or expulsed. Types of abortions include threatened, inevitable, incomplete, complete, and missed.

Risk Factors

- Chromosomal abnormalities (account for 50%)
- Maternal illness, such as type 1 diabetes mellitus
- Advancing maternal age
- Premature cervical dilation
- Chronic maternal infections
- Maternal malnutrition
- Trauma or injury
- Anomalies in the fetus or placenta
- Substance use
- Antiphospholipid syndrome

Data Collection

- Subjective and Objective Data
  - Backache, and abdominal tenderness and pain
  - Rupture of membranes, dilation of the cervix
  - Fever
  - Signs and symptoms of hemorrhage such as hypotension and tachycardia

SPONTANEOUS ABORTION (MISCARRIAGE) ASSESSMENT				
Type	Cramps	Bleeding	Tissue Passed	Cervical Opening
› Threatened	› With or without mild cramps	› Slight to spotting	› None	› Closed
› Inevitable	› Mild to severe	› Moderate	› None	› Dilated with membranes or tissue bulging at cervix
› Incomplete	› Severe	› Continuous and severe	› Partial fetal tissue or placenta	› Dilated with tissue in cervical canal or passage of tissue
› Complete	› Mild	› Minimal	› Complete expulsion of uterine contents	› Closed with no tissue in cervical canal
› Missed	› None	› Brownish discharge	› None, prolonged retention of tissue	› Closed
› Septic	› Varies	› Malodorous discharge	› Varies	› Usually dilated
› Recurrent	› Varies	› Varies	› Yes	› Usually dilated

- ○ Laboratory Tests

  - ▪ Hgb and Hct, if considerable blood loss

  - ▪ Clotting factors monitored for disseminated intravascular coagulopathy (DIC) – a complication with retained products of conception

  - ▪ WBC for suspected infection

  - ▪ Serum human chorionic gonadotropin (hCG) and progesterone levels to confirm pregnancy

- ○ Diagnostic and Therapeutic Procedures

  - ▪ Ultrasound – to determine the presence of a viable or dead fetus, or partial or complete products of conception within the uterine cavity.

  - ▪ Examination of the cervix – to observe whether it is opened or closed.

  - ▪ Dilation and curettage (D&C) – to dilate and scrape the uterine walls to remove uterine contents for inevitable and incomplete abortions.

  - ▪ Dilation and evacuation (D&E) – to dilate and evacuate uterine contents after 16 weeks of gestation.

  - ▪ Prostaglandins and oxytocin (Pitocin) – to augment or induce uterine contractions and expulse the products of conception.

Patient-Centered Care

- Nursing Actions

  - ○ Observe color and amount of bleeding (counting pads).

  - ○ Perform a pregnancy test.

  - ○ Maintain client on bed rest. Inform client of risk for falls due to sedative medications if prescribed.

  - ○ Avoid vaginal exams.

  - ○ Assist with an ultrasound.

  - ○ Administer medications, and assist with the administration of blood products.

  - ○ Determine how much tissue has passed and save passed tissue for examination.

  - ○ Assist with termination of pregnancy (D&C, D&E, prostaglandin administration) as indicated.

- Medications

  - ○ Analgesics and sedatives

  - ○ Prostaglandin – administered into the amniotic sac or as a vaginal suppository

  - ○ Oxytocin (Pitocin)

  - ○ Broad-spectrum antibiotics – in septic abortion

  - ○ Rho(D) immune globulin (RhoGAM) – suppresses immune response of clients who are Rh-negative

- Nursing Considerations

  - ○ Use the lay term "miscarriage" with clients because the medical term "abortion" can be misunderstood.

  - ○ Provide client instruction and emotional support.

  - ○ Provide referral for client and partner to pregnancy loss support groups.

- Health Promotion and Disease Prevention
  - ○ Discharge instructions
    - ▪ Provide instructions on perineal care after each voiding and bowel movement and to change perineal pads often.
    - ▪ Encourage eating foods high in iron and protein to promote tissue repair and red blood cell (RBC) replacement.
    - ▪ Recommend grief counseling/support groups.
    - ▪ Notify the provider of heavy, bright red vaginal bleeding; elevated temperature; or foul-smelling vaginal discharge.
    - ▪ A small amount of discharge is normal for 1 to 2 weeks.
    - ▪ Take prescribed antibiotics.
    - ▪ Refrain from tub baths, sexual intercourse, or placing anything into the vagina for 2 weeks.
    - ▪ Avoid becoming pregnant for 2 months.

ECTOPIC PREGNANCY

Overview

- Ectopic pregnancy is the abnormal implantation of a fertilized ovum outside of the uterine cavity usually in the fallopian tube, which can result in a tubal rupture causing a fatal hemorrhage.
- Ectopic pregnancy is the second most frequent cause of bleeding in early pregnancy and a leading cause of infertility.

Risk Factors

- Risk factors for an ectopic pregnancy include any factor that compromises tubal patency (STIs, assisted reproductive technologies, tubal surgery, and contraceptive intrauterine device [IUD]).

Data Collection

- Subjective Data
  - ○ Unilateral abdominal pain that begins as a dull, lower quadrant pain on one side. Discomfort can progress from dull pain to a colicky pain, to a sharp, stabbing pain.
  - ○ Delayed (1 to 2 weeks), lighter than usual, or irregular menses.
  - ○ Scant, dark red, or brown vaginal spotting occurs 6 to 8 weeks after last normal menses; red, vaginal bleeding if rupture has occurred.
  - ○ Referred shoulder pain due to blood in the peritoneal cavity irritating the diaphragm or phrenic nerve after tubal rupture.
  - ○ Report of faintness and dizziness related to amount of bleeding in abdominal cavity.

- Objective Data
  - Signs of hemorrhage and shock (hypotension, tachycardia, pallor)
- Laboratory Tests
  - Serum levels of progesterone greater than 25 mg/mL rules out ectopic pregnancy, and elevated hCG levels and no intrauterine pregnancy visible on ultrasound indicates an ectopic pregnancy.
- Diagnostic and Therapeutic Procedures
  - Transvaginal ultrasound showing an empty uterus
  - Caution used if vaginal and bimanual examination undertaken
  - Rapid surgical treatment
    - Salpingostomy is done to salvage the fallopian tube if not ruptured.
    - Laparoscopic salpingectomy (removal of the tube) is performed when the tube has ruptured.
    - Medical management if rupture has not occurred and tube preservation desired.
      - Methotrexate (MTX) – inhibits cell division and embryo enlargement, dissolving the pregnancy

Patient-Centered Care

- Nursing Actions
  - Replace fluids, and maintain electrolyte balance.
  - Reinforce client education and psychological support.
  - Administer medications as prescribed.
  - Prepare the client for surgery and postoperative nursing care.
  - Provide referral for client and partner to pregnancy loss support group.
- Nursing Considerations
  - Obtain serum hCG and progesterone levels, liver and renal function studies, CBC, and blood type and Rh.
- Health Promotion and Disease Prevention

  - Client education
    - Instruct the client who is prescribed methotrexate to avoid alcohol consumption and vitamins containing folic acid to prevent a toxic response to the medication.
    - Advise the client to protect herself from sun exposure (photosensitivity).

GESTATIONAL TROPHOBLASTIC DISEASE (HYDATIDIFORM MOLE, CHORIOCARCINOMA, AND MOLAR PREGNANCY)

Overview

- Gestational trophoblastic disease (GTD) is the proliferation and degeneration of trophoblastic villi in the placenta that becomes swollen, fluid-filled, and takes on the appearance of grape-like clusters. The embryo fails to develop beyond a primitive state and these structures are associated with choriocarcinoma, which is a rapidly metastasizing malignancy. Two types of molar growths are identified by chromosomal analysis.

- In the complete mole, all genetic material is paternally derived.
  - The ovum has no genetic material or the material is inactive.
  - The complete mole contains no fetus, placenta, amniotic membranes, or fluid.
  - There is no placenta to receive maternal blood. Therefore, hemorrhage into the uterine cavity occurs and vaginal bleeding results.
  - Approximately 20% of complete moles progress toward a choriocarcinoma.

- In the partial mole, genetic material is derived both maternally and paternally.
  - A normal ovum is fertilized by two sperm, or one sperm in which meiosis, or chromosome reduction and division, did not occur.
  - A partial mole often contains abnormal embryonic or fetal parts, an amniotic sac, and fetal blood, but congenital anomalies are present.
  - Approximately 6% of partial moles progress toward a choriocarcinoma.

Risk Factors

- Low carotene or animal fat intake
- Age – early teens or over age 40
- Ovulation stimulation with clomiphene (Clomid)

Data Collection

- Subjective Data
  - Excessive vomiting (hyperemesis gravidarum) due to elevated hCG levels
- Objective Data
  - Physical findings
    - Rapid uterine growth more than expected for the duration of the pregnancy due to the overproliferation of trophoblastic cells.
    - Bleeding is often dark brown resembling prune juice, or bright red that is either scant or profuse and continues for a few days or intermittently for a few weeks and can be accompanied by passage of vesicles.
    - Symptoms of preeclampsia that occur prior to 24 weeks of gestation.

- Laboratory Tests
  - Serum level of hCG persistently high compared with expected decline after weeks 10 to 12 of pregnancy.
- Diagnostic and Therapeutic Procedures
  - An ultrasound reveals a dense growth with characteristic vesicles, but no fetus in utero.
  - Suction curettage is done to aspirate and evacuate the mole.
  - Following mole evacuation, the client should undergo a baseline pelvic exam and ultrasound scan of the abdomen.
  - Serum hCG analysis following molar pregnancy to be done weekly until the level is normal and remains normal for 3 weeks, then monthly for 6 months up to 1 year to detect GTD.

Patient-Centered Care

- Nursing Actions
  - Monitor fundal height.
  - Monitor vaginal bleeding and discharge.
  - Monitor gastrointestinal status and appetite.
  - Monitor for signs and symptoms of preeclampsia.
  - Administer medications as prescribed.
    - Rho(D) immune globulin (RhoGAM) to the client who is Rh-negative
    - Assist with the administration of chemotherapeutic medications for findings of malignant cells indicating choriocarcinoma
  - Advise client to save clots or tissue for evaluation.
- Health Promotion and Disease Prevention
  - Client education
    - Provide client education and emotional support.
    - Offer referral for client and partner to pregnancy loss support group.
    - Instruct the client to use reliable contraception as a component of follow-up care.
    - Reinforce the importance of follow-up because of the increased risk of choriocarcinoma.

PLACENTA PREVIA

Overview

- Placenta previa occurs when the placenta abnormally implants in the lower segment of the uterus near or over the cervical os instead of attaching to the fundus. The abnormal implantation results in bleeding during the third trimester of pregnancy as the cervix begins to dilate and efface.

 View Image: Placenta Previa

- Placenta previa is classified into three types dependent on the degree to which the cervical os is covered by the placenta.
  - Complete or total – the cervical os is completely covered by the placental attachment
  - Incomplete or partial – the cervical os is only partially covered by the placental attachment
  - Marginal or low-lying – the placenta is attached in the lower uterine segment but does not reach the cervical os

Risk Factors

- Previous placenta previa
- Uterine scarring (previous cesarean birth, curettage, endometritis)
- Maternal age greater than 35 to 40 years
- Multifetal gestation
- Multiple gestations or closely spaced pregnancies
- Smoking

Data Collection

- Subjective Data
  - Painless, bright red vaginal bleeding during the second or third trimester
- Objective Data
  - Uterus soft, relaxed and nontender with normal tone
  - Fundal height greater than usually expected for gestational age
  - Fetus in a breech, oblique, or transverse position
  - Reassuring FHR
  - Vital signs within normal limits
  - Decreasing urinary output can be a better indicator of blood loss

- Laboratory Tests
  - Hgb and Hct for blood loss assessment
  - CBC
  - Blood type and Rh
  - Coagulation profile
  - Kleihauer-Betke test (used to detect fetal blood in maternal circulation)
- Diagnostic Procedures
  - Transabdominal or transvaginal ultrasound for placement of the placenta
  - Fetal monitoring for fetal well-being assessment

Patient-Centered Care

- Nursing Actions
  - Monitor for bleeding, leakage, or contractions.
  - Monitor fundal height.
  - Perform Leopold maneuvers (fetal position and presentation).
  - Refrain from performing vaginal exams (can exacerbate bleeding).
  - Assist with the administration of IV fluids, blood products, and medications.
    - Corticosteroids, such as betamethasone (Celestone), promote fetal lung maturation if delivery is anticipated (cesarean birth).
  - Have oxygen equipment available in case of fetal distress.
- Health Promotion and Disease Prevention
  - Discharge instructions
    - Bed rest
    - Nothing inserted vaginally

ABRUPTIO PLACENTA

Overview

- Abruptio placenta is the premature separation of the placenta from the uterus, which can be a partial or complete detachment. This separation occurs after 20 weeks of gestation, which is usually in the third trimester. It has significant maternal and fetal morbidity and mortality, and is a leading cause of maternal death.

 View Image: Abruptio Placenta

- Coagulation defect, such as DIC, is often associated with moderate to severe abruption.

Risk Factors

- Maternal hypertension (chronic or gestational)
- Blunt external abdominal trauma (motor-vehicle crash, maternal battering)
- Cocaine use resulting in vasoconstriction
- Previous incidents of abruptio placenta
- Cigarette smoking
- Premature rupture of membranes
- Multifetal pregnancy

Data Collection

- Subjective Data
  - Sudden onset of intense localized uterine pain with dark red vaginal bleeding
- Objective Data
  - Area of uterine tenderness can be localized or diffuse over uterus and boardlike
  - Contractions with hypertonicity
  - Fetal distress
  - Signs of hypovolemic shock
- Laboratory Tests
  - Hgb and Hct decreased
  - Coagulation factors decreased
  - Clotting defects (disseminated intravascular coagulation)
  - Cross and type match for possible blood transfusions
  - Kleihauer-Betke test (used to detect fetal blood in maternal circulation)
- Diagnostic Procedures
  - Ultrasound for fetal well-being and placental assessment
  - Biophysical profile to ascertain fetal well-being

Patient-Centered Care

- Nursing Actions
  - Palpate the uterus for tenderness and tone.
  - Monitor FHR pattern.
  - Assist with the administration of IV fluids, blood products, and medications as prescribed.
    - Corticosteroids to promote fetal lung maturity
  - Administer oxygen 8 to 10 L/min via face mask.
  - Monitor urinary output and monitor fluid balance.
- Client Education
  - Provide emotional support for the client and family.

APPLICATION EXERCISES

1. A nurse in the emergency department is caring for a client who reports abrupt, sharp, right-sided lower-quadrant abdominal pain and bright red vaginal bleeding. The client states she missed one menstrual cycle and cannot be pregnant because she has an intrauterine device. The nurse should suspect which of the following?

   A. Missed abortion

   B. Ectopic pregnancy

   C. Severe preeclampsia

   D. Hydatidiform mole

2. A nurse at an antepartum clinic is caring for a client who is at 4 months of gestation. The client reports continued nausea, vomiting, and scant prune-colored discharge. She has experienced no weight loss and has a fundal height larger than expected. Which of the following complications should the nurse suspect?

   A. Hyperemesis gravidarum

   B. Threatened abortion

   C. Hydatidiform mole

   D. Preterm labor

3. A nurse is providing care for a client who is diagnosed with a marginal abruptio placenta. The nurse is aware that which of the following findings are risk factors for developing the condition? (Select all that apply.)

   _____ A. Maternal hypertension

   _____ B. Blunt abdominal trauma

   _____ C. Cocaine use

   _____ D. Maternal age

   _____ E. Cigarette smoking

4. A nurse is providing care for a client who has a placenta previa at 32 weeks of gestation. The nurse notes that the client is actively bleeding. The nurse should anticipate that the provider will prescribe which of the following types of medications?

   A. Betamethasone (Celestone)

   B. Indomethacin (Indocin)

   C. Nifedipine (Adalat)

   D. Methylergonovine (Methergine)

5. A nurse is caring for a client who has a diagnosis of ruptured ectopic pregnancy. Which of the following is an expected finding?

    A. No alteration in menses

    B. Transvaginal ultrasound indicating a fetus in the uterus

    C. Serum progesterone greater than the expected reference range

    D. Report of severe shoulder pain

6. A nurse manager is presenting an educational program on placenta previa to a group of nurses. What should the nurse manager include in this presentation? Use the ATI Active Learning Template: Systems Disorder to complete this item to include the following sections:

    A. Description of the disorder: Describe the three types.

    B. Risk Factors: Identify three.

    C. Diagnostic Procedures: Describe two.

    D. Nursing Actions: Describe one that is contraindicated.

APPLICATION EXERCISES KEY

1. A. INCORRECT: A client who experienced a missed abortion would report brownish discharge and no pain.

    B. **CORRECT:** Manifestations of an ectopic pregnancy include unilateral lower quadrant pain with or without bleeding. Use of an IUD is a risk factor associated with this condition.

    C. INCORRECT: A client who has severe preeclampsia does not have vaginal bleeding and presents with right upper quadrant epigastric pain.

    D. INCORRECT: A client who has a hydatidiform mole usually has dark brown vaginal bleeding in the second trimester that is not accompanied by abdominal pain.

    Ⓝ NCLEX® Connection: Reduction of Risk Potential, Potential for Alterations in Body Systems

2. A. INCORRECT: A client who has hyperemesis gravidarum will have weight loss and signs of dehydration.

    B. INCORRECT: A client who has a threatened abortion would be in the first trimester and report spotting to moderate bleeding with no enlarged uterus.

    C. **CORRECT:** A client who has a hydatidiform mole exhibits increased fundal height that is inconsistent with the week of gestation, and excessive nausea and vomiting due to elevated hCG levels. Scant, dark discharge occurs in the second trimester.

    D. INCORRECT: Preterm labor presents prior to 37 weeks of gestation and is accompanied by pink-stained vaginal discharge and uterine contractions that become more regular.

    Ⓝ NCLEX® Connection: Reduction of Risk Potential, Potential for Alterations in Body Systems

3. A. **CORRECT:** Maternal hypertension is a risk factor associated with abruptio placenta.

    B. **CORRECT:** Blunt abdominal trauma is a risk factor associated with abruptio placenta.

    C. **CORRECT:** Cocaine use is a risk factor associated with abruptio placenta.

    D. INCORRECT: Maternal age is not a risk factor associated with abruptio placenta.

    E. **CORRECT:** Cigarette smoking is a risk factor associated with abruptio placenta.

    Ⓝ NCLEX® Connection: Physiological Adaptations, Alterations in Body Systems

4. A. **CORRECT:** Betamethasone (Celestone) is given to promote lung maturity if delivery is anticipated.

    B. INCORRECT: Indomethacin (Indocin) is prescribed for the client in preterm labor.

    C. INCORRECT: Nifedipine (Adalat) is prescribed for the client in preterm labor.

    D. INCORRECT: Methylergonovine (Methergine) is prescribed for the client experiencing postpartum hemorrhage.

    Ⓝ NCLEX® Connection: Pharmacological Therapies, Expected Actions/Outcomes

5. A. INCORRECT: A client experiencing a ruptured ectopic pregnancy has delayed, scant, or irregular menses.

    B. INCORRECT: A transvaginal ultrasound would indicate an empty uterus in a client who has a ruptured ectopic pregnancy.

    C. INCORRECT: A serum progesterone level lower than the expected reference range is an indication of ectopic pregnancy.

    D. **CORRECT:** A client's report of severe shoulder pain is a finding associated with a ruptured ectopic pregnancy due to the presence of blood in the abdominal cavity, which irritates the diaphragm and phrenic nerve.

    Ⓝ NCLEX® Connection: Physiological Adaptations, Alterations in Body Systems

6. *Using the ATI Active Learning Template: Systems Disorder*

    A. Description of the Disorder: Types of Placenta Previa
    - Complete or total – cervical os is covered by the placenta
    - Incomplete or partial – cervical os is only partially covered by the placenta
    - Marginal or low-lying – placenta is attached in the lower uterine segment but does not reach the cervical os

    B. Risk Factors
    - Previous placenta previa
    - Uterine scarring due to previous cesarean birth, curettage, or endometritis
    - Maternal age 35 to 40 years
    - Multifetal gestation
    - Multiple gestations or closely spaced pregnancies
    - Smoking

    C. Diagnostic procedures
    - Transabdominal or transvaginal ultrasound
    - Fetal monitoring

    D. Contraindicated Nursing Actions
    - Performing a vaginal exam

    Ⓝ NCLEX® Connection: Physiological Adaptations, Alterations in Body Systems

| UNIT 1 | ANTEPARTUM NURSING CARE |
| | SECTION: COMPLICATIONS OF PREGNANCY |

| CHAPTER 7 | Infections |

Overview

- Maternal infections during pregnancy require prompt identification and treatment by a provider. This section will explore HIV, TORCH infections, group B streptococcus ß-hemolytic, chlamydia, gonorrhea, and *Candida albicans*. Risk factors, assessment findings, and teamwork and collaboration will be discussed.

HIV/AIDS

Overview

- HIV is a retrovirus that attacks and causes destruction of T lymphocytes. It causes immunosuppression in a client. HIV is transmitted from the mother to a neonate perinatally through the placenta and postnatally through the breast milk.

- Routine laboratory testing in the early prenatal period includes testing for HIV. Early identification and treatment significantly decreases the incidence of perinatal transmission.

- Testing is recommended in the third trimester for clients who are at an increased risk, and rapid HIV testing should be done if a client is in labor and her HIV status is unknown.

- Procedures, such as amniocentesis and an episiotomy, should be avoided due to the risk of maternal blood exposure.

- Use of internal fetal monitors, vacuum extraction, and forceps during labor should be avoided because of the risk of fetal bleeding.

- Administration of injections and blood testing should not take place until the first bath is given to the newborn.

Risk Factors

- IV drug use
- Multiple sexual partners
- Bisexuality
- Maternal history of multiple STIs
- Blood transfusion (rare occurrence)

Data Collection

- Subjective Data
  - Fatigue and flulike symptoms
- Objective Data
  - Physical findings
    - Diarrhea and weight loss
    - Lymphadenopathy and rash
    - Anemia
  - Laboratory Tests
    - Obtain informed maternal consent prior to testing. Testing begins with an antibody screening test, such as enzyme immunoassay. Confirmation of positive results is confirmed by Western blot test or immunofluorescence assay.
    - Use rapid HIV antibody test (blood or urine sample) for a client in labor who has an unknown HIV status.
    - Screen the client for STIs such as gonorrhea, chlamydia, syphilis, and hepatitis B.
    - Obtain frequent viral load levels and CD4 cell counts throughout the pregnancy.

Teamwork and Collaboration

- Nursing Care
  - Provide counseling prior to and after testing.
  - Refer the client for a mental health consultation, legal assistance, and financial resources.
  - Use standard precautions.
  - Administer antiviral prophylaxis, triple-drug antiviral, or highly active antiretroviral therapy (HAART) as prescribed.
  - Obtain prescribed laboratory testing.
  - Encourage vaccination against hepatitis B, pneumococcal infection, *Haemophilus influenzae* type B, and viral influenza.
  - Encourage use of condoms to minimize exposure if partner is the source of infection.
  - Review plan for scheduled cesarean birth at 38 weeks for maternal viral load of more than 1,000 copies/mL.
  - Infant should be bathed after birth before remaining with the mother.
- Medications
  - Retrovir (Zidovudine)
    - Antiretroviral agent
    - Nucleoside reverse transcriptase inhibitor
  - Nursing considerations
    - Assist with the administration of retrovir at 14 weeks of gestation, throughout the pregnancy, before the onset of labor, during labor, or before cesarean birth.
    - Administer retrovir to the infant at delivery and for 6 weeks following birth.

**Q
PCC**

- Health Promotion and Disease Prevention
  - Discharge instructions
    - Instruct the client not to breastfeed.
    - Discuss HIV and safe sexual relations with the client.
    - Refer client and infant to providers specializing in the care of clients who have HIV.

TORCH INFECTIONS

Overview

- TORCH is an acronym for a group of infections that can negatively affect a woman who is pregnant. These infections can cross the placenta and have teratogenic affects on the fetus. TORCH does not include all the major infections that present risks to the mother and fetus.

Risk Factors

- Toxoplasmosis is caused by consumption of raw or undercooked meat or handling cat feces. The symptoms are similar to influenza or lymphadenopathy. Other infections can include hepatitis A and B, syphilis, mumps, parvovirus B19, and varicella-zoster. These are some of the most common and can be associated with congenital anomalies.
- Rubella (German measles) is contracted through children who have rashes or neonates who are born to mothers who had rubella during pregnancy.
- Cytomegalovirus (member of herpes virus family) is transmitted by droplet infection from person to person, and is found in semen, cervical and vaginal secretions, breast milk, placental tissue, urine, feces, and blood. A latent virus can be reactivated and cause disease to the fetus in utero or during passage through the birth canal.
- The herpes simplex virus (HSV) is spread by direct contact with oral or genital lesions. Transmission to the fetus is greatest during vaginal birth if the woman has active lesions.

Data Collection

- Subjective Data
  - Toxoplasmosis findings similar to influenza or lymphadenopathy
  - Malaise, muscle aches, (flulike symptoms)
  - Rubella joint and muscle pain
  - Cytomegalovirus has asymptomatic or mononucleosis-like manifestations

- Objective Data
  - Physical findings
    - Manifestations of toxoplasmosis include fever and tender lymph nodes.
    - Manifestations of rubella include rash, muscle aches, joint pain, mild lymphedema, fever, and fetal consequences, which include miscarriage, congenital anomalies, and death.
    - Herpes simplex virus initially presents with lesions and tender lymph nodes. Fetal consequences include miscarriage, preterm labor, and intrauterine growth restriction.
  - Laboratory Tests
    - For herpes simplex, assist with obtaining cultures from women who have HSV or are at or near term.
  - Diagnostic Procedures
    - A TORCH screen is an immunologic survey used to identify the existence of these infections in the mother (to identify fetal risks) or in her newborn (detection of antibodies against infections).
    - Prenatal screenings

Teamwork and Collaboration

- Nursing Care
  - Monitor fetal well-being.
  - Educate the client on prevention practices, including correct hand hygiene and cooking meat properly. Clients should be instructed to avoid contact with contaminated cat litter.
- Medications
  - Administer antibiotics.
  - Treatment of toxoplasmosis includes sulfonamides or a combination of pyrimethamine and sulfadiazine (potentially harmful to the fetus, but parasitic treatment is essential).
- Health Promotion and Disease Prevention
  - Client Education
    - For rubella, vaccination of women who are pregnant is contraindicated because rubella infection can develop. These women should avoid crowds of young children. Women who have low titers prior to pregnancy should receive vaccination and be instructed to use contraception for at least 1 month after receiving the vaccination.
    - Because no treatment for cytomegalovirus exists, tell the client to prevent exposure by frequent hand hygiene before eating and avoiding crowds of young children.
    - Emphasize to the client the importance of compliance with prescribed treatment.
    - Provide client with emotional support.

GROUP B, STREPTOCOCCUS ß-HEMOLYTIC

Overview

- Group B streptococcus ß-hemolytic (GBS) is a bacterial infection that can be passed to a fetus during labor and delivery.

Risk Factors

- History of positive culture with previous pregnancy
- Risk factors for early-onset neonatal GBS
  - Maternal age less than 20 years
  - African American or Hispanic ethnicity
  - Positive culture with pregnancy
  - Prolonged rupture of membranes
  - Preterm delivery
  - Low birth weight
  - Use of intrauterine fetal monitoring
  - Intrapartum maternal fever (38° C [100.4° F])

Data Collection

- Objective Data
  - Physical Findings
    - Positive GBS can have maternal and fetal effects, including premature rupture of membranes, preterm labor and delivery, chorioamnionitis, infections of the urinary tract, and maternal sepsis.
  - Laboratory Tests
    - Vaginal and rectal cultures are performed at 36 to 37 weeks of gestation.

Teamwork and Collaboration

- Nursing Care
  - Administer intrapartum antibiotic prophylaxis (IAP).
    - Client who delivered previous infant with GBS infection
    - Client who has GBS bacteriuria during current pregnancy
    - Client who has a GBS-positive screening during current pregnancy
    - Client who has unknown GBS status who is delivering at less than 37 weeks of gestation
    - Client who has maternal fever of 38° C (100.4° F)
    - Client who has rupture of membranes for 18 hr or longer

- Medications
  - Penicillin G or ampicillin (Principen) is prescribed most commonly for GBS.
    - Assist with the administration of penicillin 5 million units initially IV bolus, followed by 2.5 million units intermittent IV bolus every 4 hr during labor. The client can be prescribed ampicillin 2 grams IV initially, followed by 1 g every 4 hr.
    - Bactericidal antibiotic is used to destroy the GBS.
- Health Promotion and Disease Prevention
  - Client Education
    - Instruct the client to notify the labor and delivery nurse of GBS status.

CHLAMYDIA

Overview

- Chlamydia is a bacterial infection caused by *Chlamydia trachomatis*. It is the most common STI. The infection is often difficult to diagnose because it is typically asymptomatic. According to current guidelines from the Centers for Disease Control and Prevention, all women and adolescents ages 25 or younger who are sexually active should be screened for STIs.

Risk Factors

- Multiple sexual partners
- Unprotected sexual practices

Data Collection

- Subjective Data
  - Vaginal spotting
  - Vulvar itching
  - Postcoital bleeding and dysuria
- Objective Data
  - Physical Findings
    - White, watery vaginal discharge
  - Laboratory Tests
    - Endocervical culture

Teamwork and Collaboration

- Nursing Care
    - Instruct the client to take the entire prescription as prescribed.
    - Identify and treat all sexual partners.
    - Clients who are pregnant should be retested 3 weeks after completing the prescribed regimen.
- Medications
    - Azithromycin (Zithromax) and amoxicillin (Amoxil) are prescribed during pregnancy.
        - Broad-spectrum antibiotic
        - Bactericidal action
        - Nursing Care
            - Administer erythromycin (Romycin) to all infants following delivery. This is the medication of choice for ophthalmia neonatorum. This antibiotic is both bacteriostatic and bactericidal, so it provides prophylaxis against *Neisseria gonorrhoeae* and *Chlamydia trachomatis*.
        - Client Education
            - Instruct the client to take all prescriptions as prescribed.
            - Inform the client about the possibility of decreasing effectiveness of oral contraceptives.

GONORRHEA

Overview

- *Neisseria gonorrhoeae* is the causative agent of gonorrhea. Gonorrhea is a bacterial infection that is primarily spread by genital-to-genital contact, but also can be spread by anal-to-genital or oral-to-genital contact. It also can be transmitted to a newborn during delivery. Women are frequently asymptomatic.

Risk Factors

- Multiple sexual partners
- Unprotected sexual practices

Data Collection

- Subjective Data (Male)
    - Urethral discharge
    - Painful urination
    - Frequency
- Subjective Data (Female)
    - Lower abdominal pain
    - Dysmenorrhea

- Objective Data – Male/Female
  - Physical Findings
    - Urethral discharge
    - Yellowish-green vaginal discharge
    - Reddened vulva and vaginal walls
    - If gonorrhea is left untreated, it can cause pelvic inflammatory disease, heart disease, and arthritis.
  - Laboratory Tests
    - Obtain cultures from the endocervix, rectum, and pharynx when indicated.

Teamwork and Collaboration

- Nursing Care
  - Reinforce client education regarding disease transmission.
  - Identify and treat all sexual partners.
- Medications
  - Ceftriaxone (Rocephin) IM and azithromycin (Zithromax) PO
    - One dose prescription
    - Broad-spectrum antibiotic
    - Bactericidal action
  - Client Education
    - Instruct the client to take entire prescription as prescribed.
    - Instruct the client to repeat the culture to assess for medication effectiveness.
    - Reinforce education with the client regarding safe sex practices.

CANDIDA ALBICANS

Overview

- A fungal infection caused by *Candida albicans*.

Risk Factors

- Diabetes mellitus
- Oral contraceptives
- Recent antibiotic treatment

Data Collection

- Subjective Data
  - Vulvar itching
- Objective Data
  - Physical Findings
    - Thick, white, lumpy, cottage cheese-like consistency to vaginal discharge
    - Vulvar redness
    - White patches on vaginal walls
    - Gray-white patches on the tongue and gums (neonate)
  - Laboratory Tests
    - Wet prep
  - Diagnostic Procedures
    - Potassium hydroxide (KOH) prep
    - Presence of hyphae and pseudohyphae indicates positive findings.

Teamwork and Collaboration

- Nursing Care
  - Medications
    - Fluconazole (Diflucan)
      - Antifungal agent
      - Fungicidal action
      - Over-the-counter treatments, such as clotrimazole (Monistat), are available to treat candidiasis. However, it is important for the provider to diagnosis candidiasis initially.
- Health Promotion and Disease Prevention
  - Client Education
    - Instruct the client to avoid tight-fitting clothing.
    - Instruct the client to wear cotton-lined underpants.
    - Instruct the client to limit wearing damp clothing.
    - Instruct the client to void before and after intercourse and avoid douching.
    - Instruct the client to increase dietary intake of yogurt with active cultures.

APPLICATION EXERCISES

1. A nurse on the obstetrical unit is admitting a client who is in labor and has a positive HIV status. The nurse should know that which of the following are contraindicated for this client? (Select all that apply.)

_____ A. Episiotomy

_____ B. Vacuum extraction

_____ C. Forceps

_____ D. Cesarean birth

_____ E. Internal fetal monitoring

2. A nurse in an antepartum clinic is providing care for a client. Which of the following clinical findings are suggestive of a TORCH infection? (Select all that apply.)

_____ A. Joint pain

_____ B. Malaise

_____ C. Rash

_____ D. Urinary frequency

_____ E. Tender lymph nodes

3. A nurse is caring for a client who has a diagnosis of gonorrhea. Which of the following medications should the nurse anticipate the provider will prescribe?

A. Ceftriaxone (Rocephin)

B. Fluconazole (Diflucan)

C. Metronidazole (Flagyl)

D. Zidovudine (Retrovir)

4. A nurse is caring for a client who is in labor. The nurse should be aware that which of the following conditions have medications that can be prescribed as prophylactic treatment during labor or immediately following delivery? (Select all that apply.)

_____ A. Gonorrhea

_____ B. Chlamydia

_____ C. HIV

_____ D. Group B streptococcus ß-hemolytic

_____ E. TORCH

5. A nurse manager in a prenatal clinic is reviewing ways to prevent a TORCH infection during pregnancy with a group of newly licensed nurses during an education program. Which of the following statements by a newly licensed nurse indicates understanding of the teaching?

    A. "Obtain a vaccination against rubella early in pregnancy."

    B. "Seek prophylactic treatment if cytomegalovirus is detected."

    C. "A woman should avoid handling dog feces."

    D. "A woman should avoid consuming undercooked meat."

6. A nurse is planning care for a client who is pregnant and positive for group B streptococcus ß-hemolytic. Use the ATI Active Learning Template: Systems Disorder to complete this item to include:

    A. Laboratory Test: Describe the test and when it is performed.

    B. Risk Factors: Describe two maternal risk factors and three fetal risk factors.

    C. Medications: Describe three clients who should receive intrapartum antibiotic prophylaxis.

APPLICATION EXERCISES KEY

1. A. **CORRECT:** An episiotomy is not recommended for a client who is HIV positive because of the risk of maternal blood exposure.

   B. **CORRECT:** Vacuum extraction during delivery is not recommended because of the risk of fetal bleeding.

   C. **CORRECT:** The use of forceps during delivery is not recommended because of the risk of fetal bleeding.

   D. INCORRECT: A cesarean birth is not contraindicated for this client.

   E. **CORRECT:** Internal fetal monitoring is not recommended because of the risk of fetal bleeding.

   (N) NCLEX® Connection: Physiological Adaptations, Alterations in Body Systems

2. A. **CORRECT:** TORCH infections are flulike in presentation, such as joint pain.

   B. **CORRECT:** TORCH infections are flulike in presentation, such as malaise.

   C. **CORRECT:** TORCH infections can include findings such as a rash.

   D. INCORRECT: Urinary frequency is not a symptom associated with a TORCH infection.

   E. **CORRECT:** TORCH infections are flulike in presentation, such as tender lymph nodes.

   (N) NCLEX® Connection: Physiological Adaptations, Alterations in Body Systems

3. A. **CORRECT:** Ceftriaxone IM or cefixime is prescribed orally once for the treatment of gonorrhea.

   B. INCORRECT: Fluconazole is used to treat candidiasis.

   C. INCORRECT: Metronidazole is used in the treatment of bacterial vaginosis and trichomoniasis.

   D. INCORRECT: Zidovudine is used to treat HIV/AIDS.

   (N) NCLEX® Connection: Pharmacological Therapies, Expected Actions/Outcomes

4. A. **CORRECT:** Erythromycin (Romycin) is administered to the infant immediately following delivery to prevent *Neisseria gonorrhoeae*.

   B. **CORRECT:** Erythromycin (Romycin) is administered to the infant immediately following delivery to prevent *Chlamydia trachomatis*.

   C. **CORRECT:** Retrovir (Zidovudine) is prescribed to the client in labor who is HIV-positive.

   D. **CORRECT:** Penicillin G or ampicillin (Principen) can be prescribed to treat positive GBS.

   E. INCORRECT: A TORCH infection can be treated during pregnancy depending upon the infection.

   (N) NCLEX® Connection: Physiological Adaptations, Alterations in Body Systems

5.   A.   INCORRECT: Vaccination against rubella is contraindicated during pregnancy due to the risk of fetal congenital anomalies.

     B.   INCORRECT: There is no treatment for cytomegalovirus.

     C.   INCORRECT: A client can contract toxoplasmosis, a TORCH infection, by handling cat feces.

     D.   **CORRECT:** A client can contract toxoplasmosis, a TORCH infection, by consuming undercooked meat.

     Ⓝ NCLEX® Connection: Physiological Adaptations, Alterations in Body Systems

6.   *Using the ATI Active Learning Template: Systems Disorder*

     A. Laboratory Test
     • Vaginal and rectal cultures performed at 36 to 37 weeks of gestation

     B. Risk Factors
     • Maternal
        ○ History of positive culture with previous pregnancy
        ○ Maternal age less than 20 years
        ○ African American or Hispanic ethnicity
     • Fetal
        ○ Positive during pregnancy
        ○ Prolonged rupture of membranes
        ○ Preterm delivery
        ○ Low birth weight
        ○ Use of intrauterine fetal monitoring
        ○ Intrapartum maternal fever (38° C [100.4° F])

     C. Medications
     • Client who delivered previous infant with GBS infection
     • Client who has GBS bacteriuria during current pregnancy
     • Client who has a GBS-positive screening during current pregnancy
     • Client who has unknown GBS status who is delivering at less than 37 weeks of gestation
     • Client who has maternal fever of 38° C (100.4° F)
     • Client who has rupture of membranes for 18 hr or longer

     Ⓝ NCLEX® Connection: Physiological Adaptations, Alterations in Body Systems

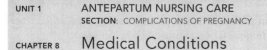

chapter 8

Overview

- Unexpected medical conditions can occur during pregnancy. Awareness, early detection, and interventions are crucial components to ensure fetal well-being and maternal health.

- Unexpected medical conditions include recurrent premature dilation of the cervix, hyperemesis gravidarum, anemia, gestational diabetes mellitus, and gestational hypertension.

RECURRENT PREMATURE DILATION OF THE CERVIX (INCOMPETENT CERVIX)

Overview

- Recurrent premature dilation of the cervix or cervical insufficiency is a variable condition whereby expulsion of the products of conception occurs. It is thought to be related to tissue changes and alterations in the length of the cervix.

Risk Factors

- History of cervical trauma (previous lacerations, excessive dilations, and curettage for biopsy), short labors, pregnancy loss in early gestation, or advanced cervical dilation at earlier weeks of gestation

- In utero exposure to diethylstilbestrol (ingested by the client's mother during pregnancy)

- Congenital structural defects of the uterus or cervix

Data Collection

- Subjective Data

  - Increase in pelvic pressure or urge to push

- Objective Data

  - Physical findings

    - Pink-stained vaginal discharge or bleeding

    - Possible gush of fluid (rupture of membranes)

    - Uterine contractions with the expulsion of the fetus

    - Postoperative (cerclage) monitoring for uterine contractions, rupture of membranes, and signs of infection

○ Diagnostic and therapeutic procedures

  ▪ An ultrasound showing a short cervix (less than 25 mm in length), the presence of cervical funneling (beaking), or effacement of the cervical os indicates reduced cervical competence.

  ▪ Prophylactic cervical cerclage is the surgical reinforcement of the cervix with a heavy ligature that is placed submucosally around the cervix to strengthen it and prevent premature cervical dilation. Best results occur if this is done before 23 to 24 weeks of gestation. The cerclage is removed at 37 weeks of gestation or when spontaneous labor occurs.

Patient-Centered Care

- Nursing Care

  ○ Evaluate the client's support systems and availability of assistance if activity restrictions and/or bed rest are prescribed.

  ○ Monitor vaginal discharge.

  ○ Monitor client reports of pressure and contractions.

  ○ Check vital signs.

- Medications

  ○ Assist with administration of tocolytics prophylactically to inhibit uterine contractions.

- Health Promotion and Disease Prevention

  ○ Discharge instructions

    ▪ Place the client on activity restriction/bed rest.

    ▪ Encourage hydration to promote a relaxed uterus. (Dehydration stimulates uterine contractions.)

    ▪ Advise the client to refrain from intercourse and to monitor for cervical/uterine changes.

  ○ Client education

    ▪ Provide client instruction about signs and symptoms to report to the provider for preterm labor, rupture of membranes, infection, strong contractions less than 5 min apart, severe perineal pressure, and an urge to push.

    ▪ Instruct the client about using the home uterine activity monitor to evaluate uterine contractions.

    ▪ Arrange for the client to follow up with a home health agency for close observation and supervision.

    ▪ Plan for removal of the cerclage around 37 weeks of gestation.

HYPEREMESIS GRAVIDARUM

Overview

- Hyperemesis gravidarum is excessive nausea and vomiting (possibly related to elevated hCG levels) that usually begins during first trimester, and 10% of clients have symptoms throughout the pregnancy. It is prolonged past 12 weeks of gestation and results in a 5% weight loss from prepregnancy weight, electrolyte imbalance, ketonuria, and ketosis.
- Hyperemesis gravidarum can be associated with altered thyroid function.
- There is a risk to the fetus for intrauterine growth restriction (IUGR) or preterm birth if the condition persists.

Risk Factors

- Maternal age younger than 20 years
- History of migraines
- Obesity
- First pregnancy
- Multifetal gestation
- Gestational trophoblastic disease or fetus with chromosomal anomaly
- Psychosocial issues and high levels of emotional stress
- Transient hyperthyroidism

Data Collection

- Objective Data
  - Physical Findings
    - Excessive vomiting for prolonged periods and diarrhea
    - Dehydration with possible electrolyte imbalance
    - Weight loss
    - Increased pulse rate
    - Decreased blood pressure
    - Poor skin turgor and dry mucous membranes
  - Laboratory Tests
    - Urinalysis for ketones and acetones (breakdown of protein and fat) is the most important initial laboratory test.
    - Elevated urine specific gravity.
    - Chemistry profile revealing electrolyte imbalances, such as:
      - Sodium, potassium, and chloride reduced from low intake
      - Acidosis resulting from excessive vomiting
      - Elevated liver enzymes
    - Thyroid test indicating hyperthyroidism.
    - Hct concentration is elevated because inability to retain fluid results in hemoconcentration.

Patient-Centered Care

- Nursing Care
  - Monitor I&O.
  - Monitor skin turgor and mucous membranes.
  - Monitor vital signs.
  - Monitor weight.
  - Have the client remain NPO for 24 to 48 hr.
  - Monitor psychosocial status.
- Medications
  - Administer IV fluids of lactated Ringer's for hydration.
  - Give pyridoxine (vitamin B_6) and other vitamin supplements as tolerated.
  - Use antiemetic medications (ondansetron [Zofran], metoclopramide [Reglan]) cautiously for uncontrollable nausea and vomiting.
  - Corticosteroids to treat refractory hyperemesis gravidarum can be prescribed, but there is little evidence that their use is effective.
- Health Promotion and Disease Prevention
  - Discharge instructions
    - Advance the client to clear liquids after 24 hr if no vomiting.
    - Advance the client's diet, as tolerated, with frequent, small meals. Start with dry toast, crackers, or cereal; then move to a soft diet; and finally to a normal diet as tolerated.
    - In severe cases, or if vomiting returns, enteral nutrition per feeding tube or total parental nutrition (TPN) can be considered.

ANEMIA

Overview

- Iron-deficiency anemia occurs during pregnancy due to inadequacy in maternal iron stores and consuming insufficient amounts of dietary iron.

Risk Factors

- Risk Factors
  - Less than 2 years between pregnancies
  - Heavy menses
  - Diet low in iron

Data Collection

- Subjective Data
  - Fatigue
  - Irritability
  - Headache
  - Shortness of breath with exertion
  - Palpitations
  - Craving unusual food (pica)
- Objective Data
  - Physical Findings
    - Pallor
    - Brittle nails
    - Shortness of breath
  - Laboratory Tests
    - Hgb less than 11 mg/dL in the first and third trimesters and less than 10.5 mg/dL in the second trimester, and a serum ferritin less than 12 mcg/dL
    - Hct less than 33%

Patient-Centered Care

- Nursing Care
  - Prophylactic treatment using prenatal supplements with 60 mg of iron is suggested.
  - Increase dietary intake of foods rich in iron (legumes, fruit, green, leafy vegetables, and meat).
  - Instruct the client about ways to minimize gastrointestinal adverse effects.
- Medications
  - Ferrous sulfate (325 mg) iron supplements twice daily
    - Nursing Considerations and Client Education
      - Instruct the client to take the supplement on an empty stomach.
      - Encourage a diet rich in vitamin C-containing foods to increase absorption.
      - Suggest that the client increase roughage and fluid intake in the diet to assist with discomforts of constipation.
  - Iron dextran (Imferon)
    - Used in the treatment of iron-deficiency anemia when oral iron supplements cannot be tolerated by the client who is pregnant.

GESTATIONAL DIABETES MELLITUS

Overview

- Gestational diabetes mellitus is an impaired tolerance to glucose with the first onset or recognition during pregnancy. The ideal blood glucose level during pregnancy should fall between 70 and 110 mg/dL.

- Symptoms of gestational diabetes mellitus can disappear a few weeks following delivery. However, approximately 50% of women will develop diabetes mellitus within 5 years.

- Gestational diabetes mellitus causes increased risks to the fetus and mother.

  ○ Spontaneous abortion, which is related to poor glycemic control

  ○ Infections (urinary and vaginal), which are related to increased glucose in the urine and decreased resistance because of altered carbohydrate metabolism

  ○ Hydramnios, which can cause overdistention of the uterus, premature rupture of membranes, preterm labor, and hemorrhage

  ○ Ketoacidosis from diabetogenic effect of pregnancy (increased insulin resistance), untreated hyperglycemia, or inappropriate insulin dosing

  ○ Hypoglycemia, which is caused by overdosing in insulin, skipped or late meals, or increased exercise

  ○ Hyperglycemia, which can cause excessive fetal growth (macrosomia)

Risk Factors

- Obesity
- Maternal age older than 25 years
- Family history of diabetes mellitus
- Previous delivery of an infant that was large or stillborn

Data Collection

- Subjective Data

  ○ Hypoglycemia (nervousness, headache, weakness, irritability, hunger, blurred vision, tingling of mouth or extremities)

  ○ Hyperglycemia (thirst, nausea, abdominal pain, frequent urination, flushed dry skin, fruity breath)

- Objective Data

  ○ Physical Findings

    ▪ Hypoglycemia

    ▪ Shaking

    ▪ Clammy pale skin

    ▪ Shallow respirations

    ▪ Rapid pulse

- Hyperglycemia
- Vomiting
- Excess weight gain during pregnancy

○ Laboratory Tests

- Routine urinalysis with glycosuria
- A glucola screening test/1-hr glucose tolerance test (50 g oral glucose load, followed by plasma glucose analysis 1 hr later performed at 24 to 28 weeks of gestation – fasting not necessary; a positive blood glucose screening is 130 to 140 mg/dL or greater; additional testing with a 3-hr oral glucose tolerance test [OGTT] is indicated)
- An OGTT (following overnight fasting, avoidance of caffeine, and abstinence from smoking for 12 hr prior to testing; a fasting glucose is obtained, a 100 g glucose load is given, and serum glucose levels are determined at 1, 2, and 3 hr following glucose ingestion)
- Presence of ketones in urine is tested to assess the severity of ketoacidosis

○ Diagnostic Procedures

- Biophysical profile to ascertain fetal well-being
- Amniocentesis with alpha-fetoprotein
- Nonstress test to assess fetal well-being

Patient-Centered Care

- Nursing Care
  ○ Monitor the client's blood glucose.
  ○ Monitor the fetus.
- Medications
  ○ Administer insulin as prescribed.
    - Most oral hypoglycemic agents are contraindicated for gestational diabetes mellitus, but there is limited use of glyburide (DiaBeta) at this time. The provider will need to determine if these medications can be used.
- Health Promotion and Disease Prevention
  ○ Client education
    - Instruct the client to perform daily kick counts.
    - Instruct the client about diet and exercise.
    - Instruct the client about self-administration of insulin.
    - Instruct the client about the need for postpartum laboratory testing to include OGTT and blood glucose levels.

GESTATIONAL HYPERTENSION

Overview

- Hypertensive disease in pregnancy is divided into clinical subsets of the disease based on end-organ effects and progresses along a continuum from mild gestational hypertension; mild and severe preeclampsia; eclampsia; and hemolysis, elevated liver enzymes, and low platelets (HELLP) syndrome.

- Vasospasm contributing to poor tissue perfusion is the underlying mechanism for the manifestations of pregnancy hypertensive disorders.

- Gestational hypertension (GH), which begins after the 20th week of pregnancy, describes hypertensive disorders of pregnancy whereby the woman has an elevated blood pressure at 140/90 mm Hg or greater recorded at least twice, 4 to 6 hr apart, and within a 1-week period. There is no proteinuria. The presence of edema is no longer considered in the definition of hypertensive disease of pregnancy. The client's blood pressure returns to baseline by 6 weeks postpartum.

- Mild preeclampsia is GH with the addition of proteinuria of greater than 1+. Report of transient headaches can occur along with episodes of irritability. Edema can be present.

- Severe preeclampsia consists of blood pressure that is 160/110 mm Hg or greater, proteinuria greater than 3+, oliguria, elevated serum creatinine greater than 1.2 mg/dL, cerebral or visual disturbances (headache and blurred vision), hyperreflexia with possible ankle clonus, pulmonary or cardiac involvement, extensive peripheral edema, hepatic dysfunction, epigastric and right upper-quadrant pain, and thrombocytopenia.

- Eclampsia is severe preeclampsia symptoms along with the onset of seizure activity or coma. Eclampsia is usually preceded by headache, severe epigastric pain, hyperreflexia, and hemoconcentrations, which are warning signs of probable convulsions.

- HELLP syndrome is a variant of GH in which hematologic conditions coexist with severe preeclampsia involving hepatic dysfunction. HELLP syndrome is diagnosed by laboratory tests, not clinically.
  - H – hemolysis resulting in anemia and jaundice
  - EL – elevated liver enzymes resulting in elevated alanine aminotransferase (ALT) or aspartate transaminase (AST), epigastric pain, and nausea and vomiting
  - LP – low platelets (less than $100,000/mm^3$), resulting in thrombocytopenia, abnormal bleeding and clotting time, bleeding gums, petechiae, and possibly disseminated intravascular coagulopathy (DIC)

- Gestational hypertensive disease and chronic hypertension can occur simultaneously.

- Gestational hypertensive diseases are associated with placental abruption, kidney failure, hepatic rupture, preterm birth, and fetal and maternal death.

Risk Factors

- No single profile identifies risks for gestational hypertensive disorders, but some high risks include the following.
  - Maternal age younger than 19 or older than 40
  - First pregnancy
  - Obesity
  - Multifetal gestation
  - Chronic renal disease
  - Chronic hypertension
  - Familiar history of preeclampsia
  - Diabetes mellitus
  - Rh incompatibility
  - Molar pregnancy
  - Previous history of GH

Data Collection

- Subjective Data
  - Severe continuous headache
  - Nausea
  - Blurring of vision
  - Flashes of lights or dots before the eyes
- Objective Data
  - Physical findings
    - Hypertension
    - Proteinuria
    - Periorbital, facial, hand, and abdominal edema
    - Pitting edema of lower extremities
    - Vomiting
    - Oliguria
    - Hyperreflexia
    - Scotoma
    - Epigastric pain
    - Right upper quadrant pain
    - Dyspnea
    - Diminished breath sounds
    - Seizures
    - Jaundice
    - Signs of progression of hypertensive disease with indications of worsening liver involvement, renal failure, worsening hypertension, cerebral involvement, and developing coagulopathies

- Abnormal Laboratory Findings
  - Elevated liver enzymes (LDH, AST)
  - Increased creatinine
  - Increased plasma uric acid
  - Thrombocytopenia
  - Decreased Hgb
  - Hyperbilirubinemia
- Laboratory Tests
  - Liver enzymes
  - Serum creatinine, BUN, uric acid, and magnesium increase as renal function decreases
  - CBC
  - Clotting studies
  - Chemistry profile
- Diagnostic Procedures
  - Dipstick testing of urine for proteinuria
  - 24-hr urine collection for protein and creatinine clearance
  - Nonstress test, contraction stress test, biophysical profile, and serial ultrasounds to assess fetal status
  - Doppler blood flow analysis to assess fetal well-being

Patient-Centered Care

- Nursing Care
  - Monitor level of consciousness.
  - Obtain pulse oximetry.
  - Monitor urine output, and obtain a clean-catch urine sample to check for proteinuria.
  - Obtain daily weights.
  - Monitor vital signs.
  - Encourage lateral positioning.
  - Perform NST and daily kick counts as prescribed.
  - Instruct the client to monitor I&O.
- Medications
  - Antihypertensive medications
    - Methyldopa (Aldomet).
    - Nifedipine (Adalat, Procardia).
    - Hydralazine (Neopresol).
    - Labetalol hydrochloride (Normodyne, Trandate).
    - Avoid ACE inhibitors and angiotensin II receptor blockers.

- ○ Anticonvulsant medications
  - Magnesium sulfate
  - Medication of choice for prophylaxis or treatment to lower blood pressure and depress the CNS
- ○ Nursing Considerations
  - Use an infusion control device to maintain a regular flow rate.
  - Inform the client that she can initially feel flushed, hot, and sedated with the magnesium sulfate bolus.
  - Monitor blood pressure, pulse, respiratory rate, deep-tendon reflexes, level of consciousness, urinary output (indwelling urinary catheter for accuracy), presence of headache, visual disturbances, epigastric pain, uterine contractions, and FHR and activity.
  - Place the client on fluid restriction of 100 to 125 mL/hr, and maintain a urinary output of 30 mL/hr or greater.
  - Monitor for signs of magnesium sulfate toxicity.
    - □ Absence of patellar deep-tendon reflexes
    - □ Urine output less than 30 mL/hr
    - □ Respirations less than 12/min
    - □ Decreased level of consciousness
    - □ Cardiac dysrhythmias
- ○ If magnesium toxicity is suspected:
  - Assist RN with immediately discontinuing infusion.
  - Assist with administration of antidote calcium gluconate.
  - Prepare for actions to prevent respiratory or cardiac arrest.
- • Health Promotion and Disease Prevention
  - ○ Discharge instructions
    - Maintain the client on bed rest, and encourage side-lying position.
    - Promote diversional activities.
    - Have the client avoid foods that are high in sodium.
    - Have the client avoid alcohol and limit caffeine.
    - Instruct the client to increase her fluid intake to 8 glasses/day.
    - Maintain a dark quiet environment to avoid stimuli that can precipitate a seizure.
    - Maintain a patent airway in the event of a seizure.
    - Administer antihypertensive medications.

APPLICATION EXERCISES

1. A nurse is caring for a client at 14 weeks of gestation who has hyperemesis gravidarum. The nurse should know that which of the following are risk factors for the client? (Select all that apply.)

_____ A. Obesity

_____ B. Multifetal pregnancy

_____ C. Maternal age greater than 40

_____ D. Migraine headache

_____ E. Oligohydramnios

2. A nurse is assisting with the administration of magnesium sulfate IV to a client who has severe preeclampsia for seizure prophylaxis. Which of the following indicates magnesium sulfate toxicity? (Select all that apply.)

_____ A. Respirations fewer than 12/min

_____ B. Urinary output less than 30 mL/hr

_____ C. Hyperreflexic deep-tendon reflexes

_____ D. Decreased level of consciousness

_____ E. Flushing and sweating

3. A nursing is caring for a client who is receiving IV magnesium sulfate. Which of the following medications should the nurse anticipate assisting with the administration of if magnesium sulfate toxicity is suspected?

A. Nifedipine (Adalat)

B. Pyridoxine (vitamin B$_6$)

C. Ferrous sulfate

D. Calcium gluconate

4. A nurse is reviewing a new prescription for ferrous sulfate with a client who is at 12 weeks of gestation. Which of the following statements by the client indicates understanding of the teaching?

A. "I will take this pill with my breakfast."

B. "I will take this medication with a glass of milk."

C. "I plan to drink more orange juice while taking this pill."

D. "I plan to add more calcium-rich foods to my diet while taking this medication."

5. A nurse is caring for a client who has suspected hyperemesis gravidarum and is reviewing the client's laboratory reports. Which of the following findings is a clinical manifestation of this condition?

    A. Hgb 12.2 g/dL

    B. Urine ketones present

    C. Alanine aminotransferase (ALT) 20 IU/L

    D. Serum glucose 114 mg/dL

6. A nurse is preparing to reinforce teaching with a client who is at 20 weeks of gestation and is to undergo a prophylactic cervical cerclage. What should be included in the instruction? Use the ATI Active Learning Template: Therapeutic Procedure to complete this item to include:

    A. Description of the Procedure

    B. Potential Complications: Identify two.

    C. Client Education: Describe at least four instructions to be given to the client.

APPLICATION EXERCISES KEY

1. A. **CORRECT:** Obesity is a risk factor for hyperemesis gravidarum.

    B. **CORRECT:** Multifetal pregnancy is a risk factor for hyperemesis gravidarum.

    C. INCORRECT: Maternal age less than 19 is a risk factor for hyperemesis gravidarum.

    D. **CORRECT:** Migraine headache is a risk factor for hyperemesis gravidarum.

    E. INCORRECT: Oligohydramnios is not a risk factor for hyperemesis gravidarum.

    (**N**) NCLEX® Connection: Physiological Adaptations, Alterations in Body Systems

2. A. **CORRECT:** A respiratory rate of less than 12/min is a sign of magnesium sulfate toxicity.

    B. **CORRECT:** Urinary output of less than 30 mL/hr is a sign of magnesium sulfate toxicity.

    C. INCORRECT: The absence of patellar deep-tendon reflexes is a sign of magnesium sulfate toxicity.

    D. **CORRECT:** Decreased level of consciousness is a sign of magnesium sulfate toxicity.

    E. INCORRECT: Flushing and sweating are adverse effects of magnesium sulfate but are not signs of toxicity.

    (**N**) NCLEX® Connection: Pharmacological Therapies, Expected Actions/Outcomes

3. A. INCORRECT: Nifedipine is an antihypertensive medication that can be administered to women who have gestational hypertension.

    B. INCORRECT: The provider can prescribe pyridoxine (vitamin B_6) a vitamin supplement for clients who have hyperemesis gravidarum.

    C. INCORRECT: Ferrous sulfate is a medication used in the treatment of iron deficiency anemia.

    D. **CORRECT:** Calcium gluconate is the antidote for magnesium sulfate.

    (**N**) NCLEX® Connection: Pharmacological Therapies, Expected Actions/Outcomes

4. A. INCORRECT: The client should take ferrous sulfate on an empty stomach.

    B. INCORRECT: Ferrous sulfate is not compatible with dairy products or juices. The client should take it with water.

    C. **CORRECT:** A diet with increased vitamin C improves the absorption of ferrous sulfate.

    D. INCORRECT: Although a diet of calcium-rich foods is appropriate for the client during pregnancy, it does not improve the effectiveness of ferrous sulfate.

    (**N**) NCLEX® Connection: Pharmacological Therapies, Expected Actions/Outcomes

5. A. INCORRECT: Altered hematocrit is a clinical manifestation of hyperemesis gravidarum because of the hemoconcentration that occurs with dehydration.

   B. **CORRECT:** The presence of ketones in the urine is associated with the breakdown of proteins and fats that occurs in a client who has hyperemesis gravidarum.

   C. INCORRECT: Liver enzymes are elevated in a client who has hyperemesis gravidarum. This finding is within the expected reference range.

   D. INCORRECT: Decreased serum glucose is anticipated in a client who has hyperemesis gravidarum. This result is within the expected reference range.

   Ⓝ NCLEX® Connection: Reduction of Risk Potential, Laboratory Values

6. *Using the ATI Active Learning Template: Therapeutic Procedure*

   A. Description of the Procedure
   - Surgical reinforcement of the cervix with a heavy ligature (suture) that is placed submucosally around the cervix to strengthen it and prevent premature cervical dilation.

   B. Potential Complications
   - Uterine contractions
   - Rupture of membranes
   - Infection

   C. Client Education
   - Remain on activity restrictions/bed rest as prescribed.
   - Increase hydration to promote a relaxed uterus.
   - Refrain from sexual intercourse.
   - Signs and symptoms to report to the provider: preterm labor, rupture of membranes, signs of infection, strong contractions less than 5 min apart, perineal pressure, and the urge to push.
   - Use of home uterine activity monitor.
   - Home health agency to follow up.
   - Plan for removal of the cerclage at 37 weeks of gestation.

   Ⓝ NCLEX® Connection: Reduction of Risk Potential, Diagnostic Tests

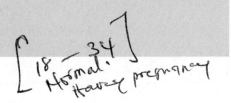

[18 - 34]
Normal:
Hearty pregnancy

Overview

- Understanding the importance of identifying the onset of early labor in a client who is pregnant is crucial for maternal and fetal well-being.

- Preterm labor, premature rupture of membranes, and preterm premature rupture of membranes are covered in this chapter.

PRETERM LABOR

Overview

- Preterm labor is defined as uterine contractions and cervical changes that occur between 20 and 37 weeks of gestation.

- It is important for a nurse to have a thorough understanding of the risk factors, examination findings, and nursing interventions to care for the client who has preterm labor.

Risk Factors

- Infections of the urinary tract, vagina, or chorioamnionitis (infection of the amniotic sac)
- Previous preterm birth
- Multifetal pregnancy
- Hydramnios (excessive amniotic fluid)
- Age below 17 or above 35
- Low socioeconomic status
- Smoking
- Substance use
- Domestic violence
- History of multiple miscarriages or abortions
- Diabetes mellitus or hypertension
- Lack of prenatal care
- Recurrent premature dilation of the cervix
- Placenta previa or abruptio placentae
- Preterm premature rupture of membranes
- Short interval between pregnancies
- Uterine abnormalities

① placenta accreta → attach → myometr
② placenta increta → invades into myometrium → tomp
③ placenta percreta → perforates through → myometr

Comp

Data Collection

- Subjective Data
  - Persistent low backache
  - Pressure in the pelvis and cramping
  - Gastrointestinal cramping, sometimes with diarrhea
  - Urinary frequency
  - Vaginal discharge
- Objective Data
  - Physical Findings
    - Increase, change, or blood in vaginal discharge
    - Change in cervical dilation
    - Regular uterine contractions with a frequency of every 10 min or greater, lasting 1 hr or longer
    - Premature rupture of membranes
  - Laboratory Tests
    - Fetal fibronectin
    - Cervical cultures
    - CBC
    - Urinalysis
  - Diagnostic Procedures
    - Monitor fetal fibronectin test. This protein is obtained by swabbing vaginal secretions and indicates when the fetal membrane integrity is lost. This test is used to determine preterm labor.
    - Measure endocervical length with an ultrasound to check for a shortened cervix, which is suggested in certain studies to precede preterm labor.
    - Use home uterine activity monitoring (HUAM), which is a uterine contraction monitor that can be used by the client at home. HUAM is not considered to be effective in preventing preterm labor.
    - Monitor cervical cultures to detect if there is a presence of infectious organisms. Culture and sensitivity results guide prescription of an appropriate antibiotic, if indicated.
    - Monitor results of a biophysical profile and/or nonstress test to provide information about the fetal well-being.

Patient-Centered Care

- Nursing Care
  - Management of a client who is in preterm labor includes focusing on stopping uterine contractions.
    - Activity restriction
      - Instruct the client on ways to modify her environment to allow for modified bed rest, yet have the ability to fulfill role responsibilities. Strict bed rest has been found to have adverse effects.
      - Encourage the client to rest in the left lateral position to increase blood flow to the uterus and decrease uterine activity.
      - Tell the client to avoid sexual intercourse.
    - Ensuring hydration
      - Dehydration stimulates the pituitary gland to secrete an antidiuretic hormone and oxytocin. Preventing dehydration prevents the release of oxytocin, which stimulates uterine contractions.
    - Identifying and treating an infection
      - Have the client report any vaginal discharge, noting color, consistency, and odor.
      - Monitor vital signs and temperature.
    - Chorioamnionitis should be suspected with the occurrence of elevated temperature and tachycardia.
    - Monitor FHR and contraction pattern.
      - Fetal tachycardia (a prolonged increase in the FHR greater than 160/min) can indicate infection, which frequently is associated with preterm labor.
- Medications
  - Nifedipine (Procardia, Adalat)
    - Classification and Therapeutic Intent
      - Nifedipine is a calcium channel blocker that is used to suppress contractions by inhibiting calcium from entering smooth muscles.
    - Nursing Considerations
      - Monitor for headache, flushing, dizziness, and nausea. These usually are related to orthostatic hypotension that occurs with administration.
      - Nifedipine should not be administered concurrently with magnesium sulfate.
    - Client Education
      - Instruct the client to slowly change positions from supine to upright and to sit until dizziness disappears.
      - Inform the client to maintain adequate hydration to counter hypotension.

- ○ Magnesium sulfate
  - ▪ Classification and Therapeutic Intent
    - □ Magnesium sulfate is a commonly used tocolytic that relaxes the smooth muscle of the uterus and thus inhibits uterine activity by suppressing contractions.
  - ▪ Nursing Considerations
    - □ Monitor the client closely. Tocolytic therapy should be discontinued immediately if the client exhibits manifestations of pulmonary edema, which include chest pain, shortness of breath, respiratory distress, audible wheezing and crackles, and a productive cough containing blood-tinged sputum.
    - □ Monitor for adverse effects.
    - □ Monitor for magnesium sulfate toxicity, and discontinue for any of the following adverse effects: loss of deep-tendon reflexes, urinary output less than 30 mL/hr, respiratory depression less than 12/min, pulmonary edema, and chest pain.
    - □ Calcium gluconate is an antidote for magnesium sulfate toxicity.
    - □ Contraindications for tocolysis include active vaginal bleeding, dilation of the cervix greater than 6 cm, chorioamnionitis, greater than 34 weeks of gestation, and acute fetal distress.
  - ▪ Client Education
    - □ Instruct the client to notify the nurse of blurred vision, headache, nausea, vomiting, or difficulty breathing.
- ○ Indomethacin (Indocin)
  - ▪ Classification and Therapeutic Intent
    - □ Indomethacin is a nonsteroidal anti-inflammatory drug (NSAID) that suppresses preterm labor by blocking the production of prostaglandins. This inhibition of prostaglandins suppresses uterine contractions.
  - ▪ Nursing Considerations
    - □ Monitor the client closely. Tocolytic therapy should be discontinued immediately if the client exhibits manifestations of pulmonary edema, which include chest pain, shortness of breath, respiratory distress, audible wheezing and crackles, and a productive cough containing blood-tinged sputum.
    - □ Indomethacin treatment should not exceed 48 hr.
    - □ Indomethacin should be used only if gestational age is less than 32 weeks.
    - □ Monitor for postpartum hemorrhage related to reduced platelet aggregation.
    - □ Administer indomethacin with food or rectally to decrease gastrointestinal distress.
    - □ Notify the provider if the client reports blurred vision, headache, nausea, vomiting, or difficulty breathing.
    - □ Monitor the neonate at birth.

- ○ Betamethasone (Celestone)
  - ▪ Classification and Therapeutic Intent
    - □ Betamethasone is a glucocorticoid that is administered IM in two injections, 24 hr apart, and requires a 24-hr period to be effective. The therapeutic action is to enhance fetal lung maturity and surfactant production.
  - ▪ Nursing Considerations
    - □ Administer the medication deep into the gluteal muscle 24 and 48 hr prior to birth of a preterm neonate.
    - □ Monitor the client and neonate for pulmonary edema by auscultating lung sounds.
    - □ Monitor for maternal and neonate hyperglycemia.
    - □ Monitor the neonate for heart rate changes.
  - ▪ Client Education
    - □ Instruct the client regarding signs of pulmonary edema (chest pain, shortness of breath, and crackles).

PREMATURE RUPTURE OF MEMBRANES
AND PRETERM PREMATURE RUPTURE OF MEMBRANES

Overview

- Premature rupture of membranes (PROM) is the spontaneous rupture of the amniotic membranes after 37 weeks of gestation prior to the onset of true labor. For most women, PROM signifies the onset of true labor if gestational duration is at term.
- Preterm premature rupture of membranes (PPROM) is the premature spontaneous rupture of membranes after 20 weeks of gestation and prior to 37 weeks of gestation.

Risk Factors

- Infection is the major risk of PROM and PPROM for both the client and the fetus. Once the amniotic membranes have ruptured, micro-organisms can ascend from the vagina into the amniotic sac. PPROM is often preceded by infection.
- Chorioamnionitis is an infection of the amniotic membranes.
  - ○ There is an increased risk of infection if there is a lag period over the 24-hr period from when the membranes rupture to delivery.

Data Collection

- Subjective Data
  - Client reports a gush or leakage of clear fluid from the vagina.
- Objective Data
  - Physical findings
    - Temperature elevation
    - Increased maternal heart rate or FHR
    - Foul-smelling fluid or vaginal discharge
    - Abdominal tenderness
  - Monitor for a prolapsed umbilical cord — *increase heart fetal*
    - Abrupt FHR variable or prolonged deceleration
    - Visible or palpable cord at the introitus
- Laboratory Tests
  - A positive Nitrazine paper test (blue, pH 6.5 to 7.5) or positive ferning test is conducted on amniotic fluid to verify rupture of membranes.

Patient-Centered Care

- Nursing Care
  - Prepare for birth if indicated.
  - Nursing management for PROM and PPROM is dependent on gestational duration, evidence of infection, or indication of fetal or maternal compromise.
  - Monitor vaginal cultures for streptococcus ß-hemolytic, chlamydia, and *Neisseria gonorrhoeae*.
  - Avoid vaginal exams.
  - Provide reassurance to reduce anxiety.
  - Obtain vital signs every 2 hr. Notify the provider of a temperature greater than 38° C (100° F).
  - Monitor FHR and uterine contractions.
  - Advise the client to adhere to bed rest with bathroom privileges.
  - Encourage hydration.
  - Obtain a CBC.
  - Instruct the client to perform daily fetal kick counts and to notify the nurse of uterine contractions.

- Medications
  - Ampicillin (Omnipen)
    - Classification and Therapeutic Intent
      - Ampicillin is an antibiotic that is used to treat infection.
    - Nursing Care
      - Monitor vaginal, urine, and blood cultures prior to administration of antibiotic.
  - Betamethasone (Celestone)
    - Classification and Therapeutic Intent
      - Betamethasone is a glucocorticoid that is administered IM in two injections, 24 hr apart, and requires a 24-hr period to be effective. The therapeutic action is to enhance fetal lung maturity and surfactant production.
      - A single dose is given with PROM at 24 to 31 weeks of gestation to reduce the risk of perinatal mortality, respiratory distress syndrome, and other morbidities.
    - Nursing Considerations
      - Administer the medication deep into the gluteal muscle 24 and 48 hr prior to birth of a preterm neonate.
      - Monitor the client and neonate for pulmonary edema by auscultating lung sounds.
      - Monitor for maternal and neonate hyperglycemia.
      - Monitor the neonate for heart rate changes.
    - Client Education
      - Instruct the client regarding signs of pulmonary edema (chest pain, shortness of breath, and crackles).
- Health Promotion and Disease Prevention
  - Discharge Instructions
    - Expect that the client will be discharged home if dilation is less than 3 cm, no evidence of infection, no contractions, and no malpresentation.
    - Advise the client to adhere to limited activity with bathroom privileges.
    - Encourage hydration.
  - Client Education for PROM and PPROM
    - The client should conduct a self-assessment for uterine contractions.
    - The client should record daily kick counts for fetal movement.
    - The client should monitor for foul-smelling vaginal discharge.
      - Refrain from inserting anything into the vagina.
    - The client should abstain from intercourse.
    - The client should avoid tub baths.
    - The client should wipe her perineal area from front to back after voiding and fecal elimination.
    - The client should take her temperature every 4 hr when awake and report a temperature that is greater than 38° C (100° F).

APPLICATION EXERCISES

1. A nurse is preparing to administer betamethasone acetate and betamethasone sodium phosphate (Celestone Soluspan) 6 mg IM to a client who will undergo a cesarean birth due to premature rupture of membranes. Available is betamethasone acetate 3 mg and betamethasone sodium phosphate 3 mg suspension per mL. How many mL should the nurse administer? (Round the answer to the nearest whole number.)

_____ mL

2. A nurse in labor and delivery is providing care for a client who is in preterm labor at 32 weeks of gestation. Which of the following medications should the nurse anticipate the provider will prescribe to hasten fetal lung maturity?

    A. Calcium gluconate

    B. Indomethacin (Indocin)

    C. Nifedipine (Procardia)

    D. Betamethasone (Celestone)

3. A nurse is caring for a client who is receiving nifedipine (Procardia) for prevention of preterm labor. The nurse should monitor the client for which of the following clinical manifestations?

    A. Blood-tinged sputum

    B. Dizziness

    C. Pallor

    D. Somnolence

4. A nurse is caring for a client who has a prescription for magnesium sulfate. The nurse should recognize that which of the following are contraindications for use of this medication. (Select all that apply.)

_____ A. Acute fetal distress

_____ B. Preterm labor

_____ C. Vaginal bleeding

_____ D. Cervical dilation greater than 6 cm

_____ E. Severe gestational hypertension

5. A nurse is reviewing discharge teaching with a client who has premature rupture of membranes at 26 weeks of gestation. Which of the following should be included in the teaching?

    A. Use a condom with sexual intercourse.

    B. Avoid bubble bath solution when taking a tub bath.

    C. Wipe from the back to front when performing perineal hygiene.

    D. Keep a daily record of fetal kick counts.

6. A nurse in a prenatal clinic is reviewing preterm labor with a newly hired nurse. What should the nurse include in the discussion? Use the ATI Active Learning Template: Systems Disorder to complete this item to include the following:

    A. Description of the Disorder.

    B. Subjective Data: Describe at least three manifestations.

    C. Objective Data: Describe at least three manifestations.

    D. Diagnostic Procedures: Describe at least three.

APPLICATION EXERCISES KEY

1. **2** mL

Using Ratio and Proportion

STEP 1: *What is the unit of measurement to calculate?*
mL

STEP 2: *What is the dose needed?*
Dose needed = Desired
6 mg

STEP 3: *What is the dose available? Dose available = Have*
3 mg

STEP 4: *Should the nurse convert the units of measurement?*
No

STEP 5: *What is the quantity of the dose available?*
1 mL

STEP 6: *Set up an equation and solve for X.*

$$\frac{Have}{Quantity} = \frac{Desired}{X}$$

$$\frac{3 \text{ mg}}{1 \text{ mL}} = \frac{6 \text{ mg}}{X \text{ mL}}$$

X = 2

STEP 7: *Round if necessary.*

STEP 8: *Reassess to determine whether the amount to give makes sense.*
If there is 3 mg/mL and the prescribed amount is 6 mg, it makes sense to give 2 mL. The nurse should administer betamethasone acetate/ betamethasone sodium phosphate suspension 2 mL IM.

Using Desired Over Have

STEP 1: *What is the unit of measurement to calculate?*
mL

STEP 2: *What is the dose needed?*
Dose needed = Desired
6 mg

STEP 3: *What is the dose available? Dose available = Have*
3 mg

STEP 4: *Should the nurse convert the units of measurement?*
No

STEP 5: *What is the quantity of the dose available?*
1 mL

STEP 6: *Set up an equation and solve for X.*

$$\frac{Desired \times Quantity}{Have} = X$$

$$\frac{6 \text{ mg} \times 1 \text{ mL}}{3 \text{ mg}} = X \text{ mL}$$

X = 2

STEP 7: *Round if necessary.*

STEP 8: *Reassess to determine whether the amount to give makes sense.*
If there is 3 mg/mL and the prescribed amount is 6 mg, it makes sense to give 2 mL. The nurse should administer betamethasone acetate/ betamethasone sodium phosphate suspension 2 mL IM.

Using Dimensional Analysis

STEP 1: What is the unit of measurement to calculate?
mL

STEP 2: What quantity of the dose is available?
1 mL

STEP 3: What is the dose available? Dose available = Have
3 mg

STEP 4: What is the dose needed?
Dose needed = Desired
6 mg

STEP 5: Should the nurse convert the units of measurement?
No

STEP 6: Set up an equation of factors and solve for X.

$$X = \frac{Quantity}{Have} \times \frac{Conversion (Have)}{Conversion (Desired)} \times \frac{Desired}{}$$

$$X \text{ mL} = \frac{1 \text{ mL}}{3 \text{ mg}} \times \frac{6 \text{ mg}}{}$$

X = 2

STEP 7: Round if necessary.

STEP 8: Reassess to determine whether the amount to give makes sense.
If there is 3 mg/mL and the prescribed amount is 6 mg, it makes sense to give 2 mL. The nurse should administer betamethasone acetate/betamethasone sodium phosphate suspension 2 mL IM.

Ⓝ NCLEX® Connection: Pharmacological Therapies, Dosage Calculation

2. A. INCORRECT: Calcium gluconate is administered as an antidote for magnesium sulfate toxicity.

   B. INCORRECT: Indomethacin is an NSAID used to suppress preterm labor by blocking prostaglandin production.

   C. INCORRECT: Nifedipine is a calcium channel blocker used to suppress uterine contractions.

   D. **CORRECT:** Betamethasone is a glucocorticoid that is given to clients in preterm labor to hasten surfactant production.

   Ⓝ NCLEX® Connection: Pharmacological Therapies, Expected Actions/Outcomes

3. A. INCORRECT: Blood-tinged sputum production is an adverse effect associated with indomethacin (Indocin).

   B. **CORRECT:** Dizziness and lightheadedness are associated with orthostatic hypotension, which occurs when taking nifedipine.

   C. INCORRECT: Facial flushing and heat sensation are adverse effects associated with nifedipine.

   D. INCORRECT: Nervousness, jitteriness, and sleep disturbances are adverse effects associated with nifedipine.

   Ⓝ NCLEX® Connection: Pharmacological Therapies, Expected Actions/Outcomes

4. A. **CORRECT:** Acute fetal distress is a complication that is a contraindication for the use of magnesium sulfate therapy.

   B. INCORRECT: Preterm labor is an indication for the use of magnesium sulfate.

   C. **CORRECT:** Vaginal bleeding is a complication that is a contraindication for magnesium sulfate therapy.

   D. **CORRECT:** Cervical dilation greater than 6 cm is a complication that is a contraindication for magnesium sulfate therapy.

   E. INCORRECT: Severe gestational hypertension is an indiction for the use of magnesium sulfate.

   Ⓝ NCLEX® Connection: Pharmacological Therapies, Expected Actions/Outcomes

5. A. INCORRECT: The client who has ruptured membranes should not insert anything into her vagina.

    B. INCORRECT: The client should take showers and avoid tub baths.

    C. INCORRECT: The client should be instructed that this is incorrect technique when performing perineal hygiene.

    D. **CORRECT:** The client should record daily fetal kick counts.

    (N) NCLEX® Connection: Physiological Adaptations, Alterations in Body Systems

6. *Using the ATI Active Learning Template: Systems Disorder*

    A. Description of the Disorder
       • Uterine contractions and cervical changes that occur between 20 and 37 weeks of gestation.

    B. Subjective Data
       • Persistent low backache
       • Pressure in the pelvis and cramping
       • Gastrointestinal cramping, sometimes with diarrhea
       • Urinary frequency
       • Vaginal discharge

    C. Objective Data
       • Increase, change, or blood in vaginal discharge
       • Change in cervical dilation
       • Regular uterine contractions with a frequency of every 10 min or greater, lasting 1 hr or longer
       • Premature rupture of membranes

    D. Diagnostic Procedures
       • Test for fetal fibronectin
       • Ultrasound to measure endocervical length
       • Cervical culture to detect presence of infectious organisms
       • Biophysical profile
       • Nonstress test
       • Home uterine activity monitoring for uterine contractions

    (N) NCLEX® Connection: Physiological Adaptations, Alterations in Body Systems

UNIT 2　　Intrapartum Nursing Care

CHAPTERS

› Nursing Care of the Client in Labor

› Fetal Assessment During Labor

NCLEX® CONNECTIONS

When reviewing the chapters in this unit, keep in mind the relevant sections of the NCLEX® outline, in particular:

Client Needs: Health Promotion and Maintenance

› Relevant topics/tasks include:
  » Ante/Intra/Postpartum and Newborn Care
    › Assist with monitoring a client in labor.
    › Assist with fetal monitoring
  » Data Collection Techniques
    › Prepare client for physical examination.

Client Needs: Pharmacological Therapies

› Relevant topics/tasks include:
  » Adverse Effects/Contraindications/Side Effects/ Interactions
    › Monitor and document client side effects to medications.
  » Pharmacological Pain Management
    › Maintain pain control devices.

Client Needs: Basic Care and Comfort

› Relevant topics/tasks include:
  » Non-Pharmacological Comfort Interventions
    › Provide non-pharmacological measures for pain relief.

Client Needs: Physiological Adaptation

› Relevant topics/tasks include:
  » Alterations in Body Systems
    › Provide care for a client experiencing complications of pregnancy/labor and/or delivery.
  » Medical Emergencies
    › Notify primary health care provider about client unexpected response/emergency situation.

chapter 10

Overview

- Intrapartum nursing care involves caring for clients just prior to the onset of labor, during the labor process, and the immediate period after delivery of the newborn.

- The labor and birth process starts when clients experience the physiological changes that precede labor, or when the process is initiated by the provider. Care can include use of a Bishop score, cervical ripening, induction/augmentation of labor, monitoring of FHR and uterine contractions, and pain management. Clients will present to a health care facility to begin the labor process and will be discharged after the delivery of the newborn in the early postpartum period.

Cervical Ripening, Labor Induction, Labor Augmentation

- Cervical ripening increases cervical readiness for labor by either a chemical or mechanical method to promote cervical softening, dilation, and effacement.

  - Chemical agents consist of prostaglandin E_1 (misoprostol [Cytotec]) and prostaglandin E_2 (dinoprostone [Cervidil insert]), which are used to "ripen" (soften and thin) the cervix and to increase cervical readiness prior to the induction of labor.

- Induction of labor is the deliberate initiation of uterine contractions to stimulate labor before spontaneous onset to bring about birth either by chemical or mechanical means.

- Augmentation of labor is the stimulation of hypotonic contractions once labor has spontaneously begun, but progress is inadequate.

- Methods

  - Amniotomy or stripping of membranes

  - Prostaglandins applied cervically

  - Nipple stimulation to trigger the release of endogenous oxytocin

  - Administration of IV oxytocin (Pitocin)

- Indications

  - Diagnoses – Any condition in which augmentation or induction of labor is indicated

- Nursing Actions

  - Preparation of Client

    - Assist with determining the Bishop score to evaluate maternal readiness for labor.

    - Assign a numerical value of 0 to 3 for cervical dilation, cervical effacement, cervical consistency, cervical position, and presenting part station.

      - A score of 9 for clients who are nullipara and 5 or more for clients who are multipara indicates readiness for labor induction.

    - Obtain the client's consent.

    - Obtain baseline FHR, maternal vital signs, and contraction pattern.

- Ongoing Care
  - ○ Prepare clients for an amniotomy or amniotic membrane stripping.
  - ○ Assist with the care of clients receiving cervical-ripening agents, undergoing amniotomy or amniotic membrane stripping, or receiving oxytocin (Pitocin) IV infusion.
  - ○ Continue to monitor FHR and uterine activity.

Monitoring Clients During Labor

- Electronic fetal monitoring is a tool to evaluate FHR patterns. First, assist with performing Leopold's maneuvers. Then, assist clients to a semi-sitting or lateral position. Apply conductive gel to an external ultrasound transducer, and place the transducer on the client's abdomen to monitor the FHR. Place a tocotransducer over the fundus to measure uterine frequency, duration, and regularity.
- Indications
  - ○ Diagnosis – term delivery
  - ○ Client presentation
    - ▪ Premonitory signs of labor
      - □ Backache – Constant low, dull backache caused by pelvic muscle relaxation
      - □ Weight loss – 0.5 to 1 kg (1 to 3 lb) weight loss
      - □ Lightening – Fetal head descends into true pelvis about 14 days before labor; feeling that the fetus has "dropped;" easier breathing, but more pressure on bladder, resulting in urinary frequency; more pronounced in clients who are primigravida
      - □ Contractions – Begin with irregular uterine contractions (Braxton Hicks) that eventually progress in strength and regularity
      - □ Bloody show – Brownish or blood-tinged mucus discharge caused by expulsion of the cervical mucus plug resulting from the onset of cervical dilation and effacement
      - □ Energy burst – Sometimes called "nesting" response
      - □ Gastrointestinal changes – Less common; include nausea, vomiting, and indigestion
      - □ Rupture of membranes – Spontaneous rupture of membranes can initiate labor or occur anytime during labor, most commonly during the transition phase.
      - □ Labor usually occurs within 24 hr of the rupture of membranes.
      - □ Prolonged rupture of membranes greater than 24 hr before delivery of fetus can lead to an infection.
- Preprocedure
  - ○ Nursing actions
    - ▪ Assist with performing initial data collection for admission to the birthing facility.
      - □ Provide culturally competent care that respects and is compatible with the client's culture.
      - □ Conduct an admission history, review of antepartum care, and review of the birth plan.
      - □ Obtain laboratory results.
      - □ Monitor baseline fetal heart tones and uterine contraction patterns for 20 to 30 min.
      - □ Obtain maternal vital signs.

- Check the status of the amniotic membranes. Check FHR pattern immediately following the rupture of membranes. Changes in FHR pattern can indicate prolapsed umbilical cord. Note abrupt decelerations, and report them to the provider.

- Observer amniotic fluid

  □ Color should be pale to straw yellow.

  □ Odor should not be foul.

  □ Clarity should appear watery and clear.

  □ Volume is between 500 to 1,000 mL.

  □ Use nitrazine paper to test fluid to confirm that it is amniotic.

    ▸ Nitrazine tests the pH of the amniotic fluid. Deep blue (6.5 to 7.5) indicates fluid that is alkaline. A yellow fluid strip indicates slight acidity because the fluid is urine.

- Determine if client is in true labor.

CHARACTERISTICS OF TRUE VS. FALSE LABOR (BRAXTON HICKS CONTRACTIONS)	
True Labor	False Labor
› Contractions	› Contractions
» Can begin irregularly, but become regular in frequency.	» Painless, irregular frequency, and intermittent.
» Stronger, last longer, and are more frequent.	» Decrease in frequency, duration, and intensity with walking or position changes.
» Felt in lower back, radiating to abdomen.	» Felt in lower back or abdomen above umbilicus.
» Walking can increase contraction intensity.	» Often stop with sleep or comfort measures such as oral hydration or emptying of the bladder.
» Continue despite comfort measures.	
› Cervix (determined by vaginal exam)	› Cervix (determined by vaginal exam)
» Progressive change in dilation and effacement.	» No significant change in dilation or effacement.
» Moves to anterior position.	» Often remains in posterior position.
» Bloody show.	» No significant bloody show.
› Fetus	› Fetus
» Presenting part engages in pelvis.	» Presenting part is not engaged in pelvis.

- Obtain clean-catch urine samples for urinalysis to ascertain maternal:

  □ Hydration status via specific gravity.

  □ Nutritional status via ketones.

  □ Proteinuria, which is indicative of preeclampsia.

  □ Urinary tract infection via bacterial count.

  □ Beta-strep culture to check for streptococcus ß-hemolytic, group B.

- Review blood tests.

  □ Hct level

  □ ABO typing and Rh-factor if not previously done

○ Client education

  - Provide clients and families with ongoing education regarding the labor and delivery process and procedures.

- Intraprocedure
  - Nursing actions
    - Assist with performing Leopold's maneuvers.
    - Check maternal vital signs per facility protocol.
    - Check maternal temperature every 1 to 2 hr if membranes are ruptured.
    - Apply external monitoring equipment.
      - Apply the tocodynamometer (tocotransducer) to the client's abdomen over the fundus to measure uterine activity.

 View Animation: Contraction Pattern

- ▸ Duration – The time between the beginning and the end of one contraction. Duration greater than 90 seconds can cause a decrease in fetal oxygenation.
- ▸ Intensity – Strength of the contraction at its peak described as mild, moderate, or strong.
- ▸ Frequency – Time from the beginning of one contraction to the beginning of the next contraction. Interval between contractions should not be less than 60 seconds to maintain fetal oxygenation.
- ▸ Resting tone of uterine contractions – Tone of the uterine muscle between contractions.
- ▸ Apply the ultrasound transducer (external fetal monitoring [EFM] transducer) to the client's abdomen to monitor FHR patterns.
- Encourage the client to void every 2 hr to prevent bladder distention.
- Encourage the client to change positions frequently.
- Assist with a vaginal examination – Performed digitally by the provider or qualified nurse to assess for:
  - ▸ Cervical dilation (stretching of cervical os adequate to allow fetal passage) and effacement (cervical thinning and shortening).
  - ▸ Descent of the fetus through the birth canal as measured by fetal station in centimeters.
  - ▸ Fetal position, presenting part, and lie.
- Assist with monitoring clients in labor.

STAGES OF LABOR			
DURATION	**BEGINS WITH**	**ENDS WITH**	**MATERNAL CHARACTERISTICS**
FIRST STAGE			
› 12.5 hr	› Onset of labor	› Complete dilation	› Cervical dilation 1 cm/hr for clients who are primigravida, and 1.5 cm/hr for clients who are multigravida, on average
Latent Phase			
› Primigravida: 6 hr › Multigravida: 4 hr	› Cervix 0 cm › Irregular, mild to moderate contractions › Frequency 5 to 30 min › Duration 30 to 45 seconds	› Cervix 3 cm	› Some dilation and effacement › Talkative and eager
Active Phase			
› Primigravida: 3 hr › Multigravida: 2 hr	› Cervix 4 cm › More regular, moderate to strong contractions › Frequency 3 to 5 min › Duration 40 to 70 seconds	› Cervix 7 cm dilated	› Rapid dilation and effacement › Some fetal descent › Feelings of helplessness › Anxiety and restlessness increase as contractions become stronger
Transition			
› 20 to 40 min	› Cervix 8 cm › Strong to very strong contractions › Frequency 2 to 3 min › Duration 45 to 90 seconds	› Complete dilation at 10 cm	› Tired, restless, and irritable › Feeling out of control, client often states, "cannot continue" › Can have nausea and vomiting › Urge to push › Increased rectal pressure and feelings of needing to have a bowel movement › Increased bloody show › Most difficult part of labor
SECOND STAGE			
› Primigravida: 30 min to 2 hr › Multigravida: 5 to 30 min	› Full dilation › Progresses to intense contractions every 1 to 2 min	› Birth	› Pushing results in birth of fetus
THIRD STAGE			
› 5 to 30 min	› Delivery of the neonate	› Delivery of placenta	› Placental separation and expulsion › Schultze presentation: shiny fetal surface of placenta emerges first › Duncan presentation: dull maternal surface of placenta emerges first
FOURTH STAGE			
› 1 to 4 hr	› Delivery of placenta	› Maternal stabilization of vital signs	› Achievement of vital sign homeostasis › Lochia scant to moderate rubra

Monitor the fetal Heart rate (handwritten)

dixox (handwritten)

Hamrge (handwritten)

90 second will not Last (handwritten)

M View Media

› Stages of Labor (Video)   › Schultze and Dirty Duncan Placenta (Images)

- Discourage pushing efforts until the cervix is fully dilated.

- Observe for perineal bulging or crowning (appearance of the fetal head at the perineum).

- Encourage clients to begin bearing down with contractions once the cervix is fully dilated. Listen for client statements expressing the need to have a bowel movement. This sensation is a sign of complete dilation and fetal descent.

- Assist with providing pain management.

TIMING AND EFFECTIVENESS OF PAIN RELIEF MEASURES DURING LABOR				
First Stage (Latent Phase)	First Stage (Active Phase)	Transition	Second Stage	Third Stage
Nonpharmacological methods →				
Sedatives			Spinal block →	
	Opioids Epidural →			
			Pudendal →	
			Local infiltration →	

Nonpharmacological Pain Management

- Assist the client to use nonpharmacological measures to promote relaxation and relieve the discomfort of labor. These include breathing techniques, effleurage, music, massage, sacral counterpressure, hydrotherapy, and heat or cold therapy.

- Indications

  ○ Diagnosis – Term delivery

  ○ Client presentation – Client reports pain.

  ○ Nursing actions

   ▪ Assist the client with breathing techniques. Encourage deep cleansing breaths. Check for signs of hyperventilation (caused by low blood levels of PCO_2 from blowing off too much CO_2), such as lightheadedness and tingling of the fingers.

    - If hyperventilation occurs, have the client breathe into a paper bag or her cupped hands.

   ▪ Assist the client with sensory stimulation strategies to promote relaxation and pain relief.

    - Aromatherapy

    - Breathing techniques

    - Imagery

    - Music

    - Use of focal points

- Assist clients with cutaneous strategies to promote relaxation and pain relief.
  - Back rubs and massage
  - Effleurage
    - Light, gentle circular stroking of the client's abdomen with the fingertips in rhythm with breathing during contractions
  - Sacral counterpressure
    - Consistent pressure is applied by the support person using the heel of the hand or fist against the client's sacral area to counteract pain in the lower back.
  - Heat or cold therapy
  - Hydrotherapy (whirlpool or shower) increases maternal endorphin levels
  - Intradermal water block
  - Hypnosis
  - Acupressure
    - Transcutaneous electrical nerve stimulation (TENS) unit
- Promote frequent maternal position changes to promote relaxation and pain relief.
  - Semi-sitting
  - Squatting
  - Kneeling
  - Kneeling and rocking back and forth
  - Supine position only with the placement of a wedge under one of the client's hips to tilt the uterus and avoid supine hypotension syndrome

Pharmacological Pain Management

- Alleviates pain sensations or raises the threshold for pain perception
- Clients can be given IM or IV opioid analgesics as a pharmacological method of pain management. Epidural and spinal regional analgesia can be administered by an anesthesia care provider. Regional blocks, such as a pudendal block or a paracervical nerve block, can be administered by the provider to provide local anesthesia to the perineum, vulva, and rectal areas during delivery, episiotomy, and episiotomy repair.
- Indications
  - Diagnosis – Term delivery
  - Client presentation – The client reports pain.

- ○ Nursing actions
  - ▪ Opioid analgesics such as meperidine hydrochloride (Demerol), fentanyl (Sublimaze), butorphanol (Stadol), and nalbuphine act in the CNS to decrease the perception of pain without the loss of consciousness. Clients can be given opioid analgesics IM or IV, but the IV route is recommended during labor because action is quicker.
    - □ Butorphanol (Stadol) and nalbuphine provide pain relief without causing significant respiratory depression in the mother or fetus.
  - ▪ Monitor for adverse effects
    - □ Crosses the placental barrier; if given to the mother too close to the time of delivery, can cause respiratory depression in the newborn
    - □ Reduced gastric emptying; increased risk for nausea and emesis
    - □ Increased risk for aspiration of food or fluids in the stomach
    - □ Sedation
    - □ Tachycardia
    - □ Hypotension
    - □ Decreased FHR variability
    - □ Allergic reaction
  - ▪ Have naloxone (Narcan) available to counteract the effects of respiratory depression in the newborn.
    - □ Administer antiemetics.
    - □ Monitor maternal vital signs, uterine contraction pattern, and FHR.
    - □ Dim the lights, and provide a quiet atmosphere.
    - □ Provide safety for the client by lowering the position of the bed and elevate the side rails.
- ○ Client education
  - ▪ Explain to the client that the medication will cause drowsiness.
  - ▪ Instruct the client to request assistance with ambulation.
  - ▪ Phenothiazine medications such as promethazine or hydroxyzine (Vistaril) can control nausea and anxiety. They do not relieve pain and are used as an adjunct with opioids. Zofran and Reglan are antiemetics that cause little sedation and have few side effects.
- ○ Nursing actions
  - ▪ Monitor for sedation and dry mouth
    - □ Provide ice chips or mouth swabs.
    - □ Provide safety measures to clients.
- ○ Epidural and spinal regional analgesia consists of using analgesics such as fentanyl (Sublimaze) and sufentanil (Sufenta), which are short-acting opioids that are administered as a motor block into the epidural or intrathecal space without anesthesia. These opioids produce regional analgesia, providing rapid pain relief while still allowing clients to sense contractions and maintain the ability to bear down.

○ Nursing actions

- Monitor the client for adverse effects.

  □ Decreased gastric emptying resulting in nausea and vomiting

  □ Inhibition of bowel and bladder elimination sensations

  □ Bradycardia or tachycardia

  □ Hypotension

  □ Respiratory depression

  □ Allergic reaction and pruritus

- Institute safety precautions, such as putting side rails up on the client's bed. Clients can experience dizziness and sedation, which increases maternal risk for injury.

- Monitor for nausea and emesis and administer antiemetics as prescribed.

- Monitor maternal vital signs per facility protocol.

- Monitor for allergic reaction.

- Continue FHR pattern monitoring.

○ Client education

- Provide the client with ongoing instruction related to expectations for procedure.

○ Anesthesia used in childbirth includes regional blocks and general anesthesia (rarely used).

○ Regional blocks are most commonly used and consist of pudendal, epidural, spinal, and paracervical nerve block. Pharmacological anesthesia eliminates pain perceptions by interrupting the nerve impulses to the brain.

- Pudendal block consists of a local anesthetic such as lidocaine (Xylocaine) or bupivacaine (Marcaine) being administered transvaginally into the space in front of the pudendal nerve. This type of block has no maternal or fetal systemic effects, but it does provide local anesthesia to the perineum, vulva, and rectal areas during delivery, episiotomy, and episiotomy repair. It is administered during the second stage of labor 10 to 20 min before delivery, providing analgesia prior to spontaneous expulsion of the fetus or forceps- or vacuum-assisted birth.

  □ Nursing actions

    ▸ Monitor clients for adverse effects.

      ▹ Broad ligament hematoma

      ▹ Compromise of maternal bearing-down reflex

    ▸ Coach clients about when to bear down.

    ▸ Check the perineal and vulvar area postpartum for hematoma.

  □ Client education

    ▸ Provide clients with ongoing instruction related to expectations for procedure.

- An epidural block consists of a local anesthetic bupivacaine (Marcaine) along with an analgesic morphine (Duramorph) or fentanyl (Sublimaze) injected into the epidural space at the level of the fourth or fifth vertebrae. This eliminates all sensation from the level of the umbilicus to the thighs, relieving the discomfort of uterine contractions, fetal descent, and pressure and stretching of the perineum. It is administered when clients are in active labor and dilated to at least 4 cm. Continuous infusion or intermittent injections can be administered through an indwelling epidural catheter. Patient-controlled epidural analgesia is a new technique for labor analgesia and is becoming a favored method of acute pain relief management for labor and birth.

  □ Nursing actions

    ▸ Monitor for adverse effects.

      ▷ Maternal hypotension

      ▷ Fetal bradycardia

      ▷ Inability to feel the urge to void

      ▷ Loss of the bearing-down reflex

    ▸ Monitor the client receiving a bolus of IV fluids to help offset maternal hypotension.

    ▸ Help to position and steady the client into either a sitting or side-lying modified Sims' position, with the client's back curved to widen the intervertebral space for insertion of the epidural catheter.

    ▸ Encourage the client to remain in the side-lying position after insertion of the epidural catheter to avoid supine hypotension syndrome with compression of the vena cava.

    ▸ Coach the client in pushing efforts, and request an evaluation of epidural pain management by anesthesia if pushing efforts are ineffective.

    ▸ Monitor maternal blood pressure and pulse. Observe for hypotension, respiratory depression, and oxygen saturations.

    ▸ Monitor FHR patterns continuously.

    ▸ Ensure oxygen and suction equipment is available.

    ▸ Provide client safety such as raising the side rails of the bed. Do not allow the client to ambulate unassisted until all motor control has returned.

    ▸ Check the maternal bladder for distention at frequent intervals and catheterize if necessary to assist with voiding.

    ▸ Monitor for the return of sensation in the client's legs after delivery but prior to standing. Assist the client with standing and walking for the first time after a delivery that included epidural anesthesia.

  □ Client education

    ▸ Provide ongoing instructions related to the procedure and nursing actions.

- Spinal block consists of a local anesthetic that is injected into the subarachnoid space into the spinal fluid at the third, fourth, or fifth lumbar interspace. This can be done alone or in combination with an analgesic such as fentanyl (Sublimaze). The spinal block eliminates all sensations from the level of the nipples to the feet. It is used commonly for cesarean births. A low spinal block can be used for a vaginal birth, but is not used for labor. A spinal block is administered in the late second stage or before cesarean birth.

  □ Nursing actions

    ▸ Monitor for adverse effects.

      ▹ Maternal hypotension

      ▹ Fetal bradycardia

      ▹ Loss of the bearing-down reflex in the mother with a higher incidence of operative births

      ▹ Potential headache from leakage of cerebrospinal fluid at the puncture site

      ▹ Bladder and uterine atony following birth

    ▸ Check maternal vital signs per facility protocol.

    ▸ Monitor FHR patterns continuously.

    ▸ Provide client safety to prevent injury by raising the side rails of the bed and assisting the client with repositioning and ambulating.

    ▸ Encourage interventions to relieve a postpartum headache resulting from a cerebrospinal fluid leak. Interventions include placing the client in a supine position; promoting bed rest in a dark room; and administering oral analgesics, caffeine, and fluids. An autologous blood patch is the most beneficial and reliable relief measure for cerebrospinal fluid leaks.

  □ Client education

    ▸ Instruct clients about the method.

- Postprocedure

  ○ Nursing actions

    - Check maternal vital signs every 15 min for the first hour and then according to facility protocol.

    - Check fundus and lochia every 15 min for the first hour and then according to facility protocol.

    - Massage the uterine fundus and/or administer oxytocics to maintain uterine tone and to prevent hemorrhage.

    - Encourage voiding to prevent bladder distention.

    - Promote an opportunity for maternal-infant bonding.

- Complications

  ○ Fetal distress

    - Indications

      □ FHR less than 110/min or greater than 160/min.

      □ FHR shows decreased or no variability.

      □ Fetal hyperactivity or no fetal activity.

      □ Fetal blood pH less than 7.2.

- ○ Nursing actions
  - ▪ Notify the provider.
  - ▪ Assist the charge nurse to:
    - □ Position clients in a side-lying reclining position with legs elevated to increase uteroplacental perfusion.
    - □ Administer 8 to 10 L/min of oxygen via a face mask.
    - □ Maintain IV infusion at 200 mL/min or as prescribed.
    - □ Prepare the client for an emergency cesarean birth.
- ○ Client education
  - ▪ Provide support to the client and her family.
- • Prolapsed cord
  - ○ A prolapsed umbilical cord occurs when the umbilical cord is displaced, preceding the presenting part of the fetus, or protruding through the cervix. Visualization or palpation of the umbilical cord protruding from the introitus results in cord compression and compromised fetal circulation. Extreme increase in fetal activity that occurs and then ceases is suggestive of severe fetal hypoxia. Risk factors include transverse lie, multifetal pregnancy, cephalopelvic disproportion, an unusually long umbilical cord, and hydramnios.
  - ○ Nursing actions
    - ▪ Call for assistance immediately.
    - ▪ Have another nurse notify the provider immediately.
    - ▪ Use a sterile-gloved hand, insert two fingers into the vagina, and apply finger pressure on either side of the cord to the fetal presenting part to elevate it off of the cord.
    - ▪ Place a rolled towel under the client's hip to relieve pressure on the cord.
    - ▪ Reposition the client in a knee-chest, Trendelenburg, or a side-lying position.
    - ▪ Apply a sterile, saline-soaked towel to the cord to prevent drying and to maintain blood flow if the cord is protruding from the vaginal introitus.
    - ▪ Assist the charge nurse to:
      - □ Monitor the FHR.
      - □ Administer oxygen at 8 to 10 L/min via a face mask. This will improve fetal oxygenation.
      - □ Assist with initiating IV infusion or assist with administering a bolus.
      - □ Prepare the client for a cesarean birth.
  - ○ Client education
    - ▪ Provide support to the client and her families.

APPLICATION EXERCISES

1. A client reports that her contractions started about 1 hr ago and decreased after drinking two glasses of water and walking. She reports that contractions occur every 10 to 15 min and that she hasn't had any fluid leaking or vaginal bleeding. The nurse should recognize that the client is experiencing which of the following?

   A. Braxton Hicks contractions

   B. Rupture of membranes

   C. Fetal descent

   D. True contractions

2. While the nurse is assisting with an admission history for a client at 39 weeks of gestation, the client tells the nurse that water has been leaking from her vagina for 2 days. The nurse should know that this client is at risk for which of the following?

   A. Cord prolapse

   B. Infection

   C. Postpartum hemorrhage

   D. Hydramnios

3. A nurse is reinforcing nonpharmacologic pain interventions for lower back pain due to occiput posterior presentation with a group of clients. Which of the following statements regarding nonpharmacologic interventions indicates the client understands an effective intervention for this type of pain?

   A. "I should use effleurage to alleviate the discomfort."

   B. "I will get my husband to apply sacral counterpressure during labor."

   C. "I will try hydrotherapy during my labor to relieve the back pain."

   D. "I should use massage throughout my labor."

4. A nurse is assisting with the care of a client who is primipara and active labor who received meperidine (Demerol) 50 mg IV bolus for pain 30 min prior to precipitous delivery. The nurse should know that naloxone (Narcan) is to be administered to the newborn for which of the following?

   A. Hypoglycemia

   B. Hyperbilirubinemia

   C. Respiratory depression

   D. Maternal substance use disorder

5. A nurse is assisting with the management of a client who is in active labor. Which of the following findings should the nurse report following epidural placement?

    A. Blood pressure 89/54 mm Hg

    B. 2+ pedal edema

    C. Early decelerations

    D. Fetal heart rate 160

6. The manager of a labor and delivery unit is reviewing the procedure for vaginal examination with a group of newly hired nurses. Which of the following interventions should be included in this discussion? Use the ATI Active Learning Template: Therapeutic Procedure to complete this item to include the following:

    A. Nursing Actions: Describe four actions that are preprocedure, intraprocedure, and postprocedure.

    B. Describe three data collection findings that can be determined by the procedure.

APPLICATION EXERCISES KEY

1. A. **CORRECT:** Braxton Hicks contractions decrease with hydration and walking.

   B. INCORRECT: Rupture of membranes is when the amniotic membranes rupture and allows the amniotic fluid to escape.

   C. INCORRECT: Fetal descent is the downward movement of the fetus in the birth canal.

   D. INCORRECT: True contractions do not go away with hydration or walking. They are regular in frequency, duration, and intensity, and become stronger with walking.

   (N) NCLEX® Connection: Health Promotion and Maintenance, Ante/Intra/Postpartum and Newborn Care

2. A. INCORRECT: Cord prolapse is a risk with rupture of membranes. However, it occurs when the fluid rushes out rather than trickling or leaking out.

   B. **CORRECT:** Rupture of membranes exceeding 24 hr before delivery increases the risk of infectious organisms entering vaginally into the uterus.

   C. INCORRECT: This client is not at an increased risk vs. other pregnant clients for postpartum hemorrhage.

   D. INCORRECT: The client is more likely to have oligohydramnios or insufficient amniotic fluid.

   (N) NCLEX® Connection: Physiological Adaptations, Alterations in Body Systems

3. A. INCORRECT: Abdominal effleurage is a gentle stroking of the abdomen in rhythm with breathing during contractions.

   B. **CORRECT:** Sacral counterpressure is the application of steady pressure to the lower back to counteract the pressure exerted on the spinal nerves by the fetus, which especially occurs with an occiput posterior presentation.

   C. INCORRECT: Hydrotherapy can be helpful, but counterpressure is the most effective in relieving back discomfort.

   D. INCORRECT: Massage can be helpful, but counterpressure is the most effective in relieving back discomfort.

   (N) NCLEX® Connection: Basic Care and Comfort, Non-Pharmacological Comfort Interventions

4. A. INCORRECT: Hypoglycemia is not an indication for naloxone administration.

    B. INCORRECT: Hyperbilirubinemia is not an indication for naloxone administration.

    C. **CORRECT:** Naloxone (Narcan) is an opioid antagonist that should be administered to the newborn for respiratory depression.

    D. INCORRECT: Maternal substance use disorder is not an indication for naloxone administration.

    (N) NCLEX® Connection: Pharmacological Therapies, Adverse Effects/Contraindications/Side Effects/ Interactions

5. A. **CORRECT:** The nurse should monitor the client for hypotension and report this if it occurs following epidural placement because it is an adverse effect of epidural placement.

    B. INCORRECT: Epidural placement has no effect on maternal edema.

    C. INCORRECT: Early decelerations are common as labor progresses.

    D. INCORRECT: Fetal heart rate of 160/min is within the expected range.

    (N) NCLEX® Connection: Pharmacological Therapies, Pharmacological Pain Management

6. *Using the ATI Active Learning Template: Therapeutic Procedure*

    A. Nursing Actions
    • Explain the procedure, and assist with obtaining the client's permission for the examination.
    • Don sterile gloves with antiseptic solution or soluble gel for lubrication.
    • Position the client to avoid supine hypotension.
    • Provide for privacy.
    • Cleanse the vulva or perineum if needed.
    • Insert the index and middle fingers into the client's vagina.
    • Explain findings to the client.
    • Document findings, and report to the provider.

    B. Data Collection Findings
    • Cervical dilation, effacement, and position
    • Fetal presenting part, position, and station
    • Status of membranes
    • Characteristics of amniotic fluid if membranes ruptured

    (N) NCLEX® Connection: Health Promotion and Maintenance, Data Collection Techniques

chapter 11

Overview

- Describe fetal assessment during labor.
- The diagnostic procedures mentioned in this chapter include FHR pattern and uterine contraction monitoring, Leopold maneuvers, fetal scalp blood sampling, and fetal oxygen monitoring.

LEOPOLD MANEUVERS

- Description of Procedure
  - Leopold maneuvers consist of performing external palpations of the maternal uterus through the abdominal wall.
- Indications
  - To determine:
    - Number of fetuses – one, two, or more fetuses
    - Presenting part, fetal lie, and fetal attitude
    - Expected location of the point of maximal impulse (PMI)
      - PMI is the optimal location where the fetal heart tones are auscultated the loudest on the woman's abdomen. These tones are best heard directly over the fetal back.
      - In vertex presentation, PMI is either in the right- or left-lower quadrant or below the maternal umbilicus.
      - In breech presentation, PMI is either in the right- or left-upper quadrant above the maternal umbilicus.
- Nursing Actions
  - Preparation of the client
    - Ask the client to empty her bladder before beginning the assessment.
    - Place the client in the supine position with a pillow under her head and have her flex her knees slightly.
    - Place a wedge under her right hip to displace the uterus to the left and prevent supine hypotension/vena cava syndrome.
  - Ongoing care
    - Identify the fetal part occupying the fundus. The head should feel round and firm, and move freely. A breech position should feel irregular and soft.
    - Identify the fetal lie and presenting part.

- Locate and palpate the smooth contour of the fetal back using the palm of one hand and the irregular small parts of the hands, feet, and elbows using the palm of the other hand. This maneuver validates the presenting part.

- Determine the fetal presenting part over the true pelvis inlet by gently grasping the lower segment of the uterus between the thumb and fingers. If the head is presenting and not engaged, determine whether the head is flexed or extended. This maneuver assists in identifying the descent of the presenting part into the pelvis.

- Face the client's feet and outline the fetal head using the palmar surface of the fingertips on both hands to palpate the cephalic prominence. If the cephalic prominence is on the same side as the small parts, the head is flexed with vertex presentation. If the cephalic prominence is on the same side as the back, the head is extended with a face presentation. This maneuver identifies the fetal attitude.

○ Interventions

- Auscultate the FHR postmaneuvers to determine the fetal tolerance to the procedure.

- Document the findings from the maneuvers.

FHR PATTERN AND UTERINE CONTRACTION MONITORING

- Description of Procedure

○ Intermittent auscultation and uterine contraction palpation

- Intermittent auscultation of the FHR is a low-technology method that can be performed during labor using a handheld Doppler ultrasound device, ultrasound stethoscope, or fetoscope to check FHR. In conjunction, palpation of contractions at the fundus for frequency, duration, and intensity is used to evaluate fetal well-being. During labor, uterine contractions compress the uteroplacental arteries, temporarily stopping maternal blood flow into the uterus and intervillous spaces of the placenta, decreasing fetal circulation and oxygenation. Circulation to the uterus and placenta resumes during uterine relaxation between contractions. For low-risk labor and delivery, this procedure allows the woman freedom of movement and can be done at home or a birthing center.

- Follow the facility's policy regarding intermittent auscultation or continuous electronic fetal monitoring.

- Indications

○ Potential diagnoses

- Rule out labor

- Active labor

○ Guidelines for intermittent auscultation following routine procedures

- Rupture of membranes, either spontaneously or artificially

- Preceding and subsequent to ambulation

- Prior to and following administration of or a change in medication anesthesia

- At peak action of anesthesia

- Following vaginal examination

- Following expulsion of an enema
- After urinary catheterization
- In the event of abnormal or excessive uterine contractions

- Interpretation of Findings
  - A normal, reassuring FHR is 110 to 160/min with increases and decreases from baseline.
- Nursing Actions
  - Preparation of the client
    - Perform Leopold maneuvers to determine point of maximum impulse (PMI).
    - Auscultate at PMI using listening device.
    - Palpate the client's abdomen at uterine fundus to determine uterine activity.
    - Count FHR for 30 to 60 seconds to determine baseline rate.
    - Auscultate FHR during a contraction and for 30 seconds following the completion of the contraction.
  - Ongoing care
    - Identify any nonreassuring FHR patterns and notify the provider.
  - Interventions
    - It is the responsibility of the nurse to evaluate FHR patterns, implement nursing interventions, and report nonreassuring patterns to the provider.

    - The cultural considerations, emotional, educational, and comfort needs of the mother and the family must be incorporated into the plan of care while continuing to determine the FHR pattern's response to the labor process.
  - The method and frequency of fetal surveillance during labor will vary and depend on maternal-fetal risk factors as well as the preference of the facility, provider, and client.
- Description of Procedure
  - Continuous electronic fetal monitoring
    - Continuous external fetal monitoring is accomplished by securing an ultrasound transducer over the client's abdomen to determine PMI, which records the FHR pattern, and a tocotransducer on the fundus that records the uterine contractions.
  - Advantages of external fetal monitoring
    - Noninvasive and reduces risk for infection.
    - Membranes do not have to be ruptured.
    - Cervix does not have to be dilated.
    - Placement of transducers can be performed by the nurse.
    - Records permanent record of FHR tracing.
  - Disadvantages of external fetal monitoring
    - Contraction intensity is not measurable.
    - Movement of the client requires frequent 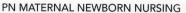 repositioning of transducers.
    - Quality of recording is affected by client obesity and fetal position.

- Indications for Monitoring *ice — prevent ① pain ② swelling*
  - Potential diagnoses
    - Multiple gestations; oxytocin (Pitocin) infusion (augmentation or induction of labor)
    - Placenta previa *— delivery on C-Section x or put her woman Bed rest.*
    - Fetal bradycardia
    - Maternal complications (diabetes mellitus, gestational hypertension, kidney disease)
    - Intrauterine growth restriction
    - Post date
    - Active labor
    - Meconium-stained amniotic fluid
    - Abruptio placentae – suspected or actual *✓ before the baby birth this is pain, hardness, rigid*
    - Abnormal nonstress test or contraction stress test
    - Abnormal uterine contractions
    - Fetal distress
  - Interpretation of findings
    - A normal fetal heart rate baseline at term is 110 to 160/min excluding accelerations, decelerations, and periods of marked variability within a 10 min window. At least 2 min of baseline segments in a 10-min window should be present. A single number should be documented instead of a baseline range.
    - Fetal heart rate baseline variability is described as fluctuations in the FHR baseline that are irregular in frequency and amplitude. Classification of variability is as follows:
      - Absent or undetectable variability (considered nonreassuring)
      - Minimal variability (greater than undetectable but less than 5/min)
      - Moderate variability (6 to 25/min)
      - Marked variability (greater than 25/min)
    - Changes in fetal heart rate patterns are categorized as episodic or periodic changes. Episodic changes are not associated with uterine contractions and periodic changes occur with uterine contractions. These changes include accelerations and decelerations.
    - According to a report from the 2008 National Institute of Child Health Human Development Workshop, current recommendations for fetal monitoring include a three-tier fetal heart rate interpretation system.
      - Category I – All of the following are included in the fetal heart rate tracing:
        - Baseline fetal heart rate of 110 to 160/min
        - Baseline fetal heart rate variability – Moderate
        - Accelerations – Present or absent
        - Early decelerations – Present or absent
        - Variable or late decelerations – Absent

- Category II – Category II tracings include all fetal heart rate tracings not categorized as Category I or Category III. Examples of Category II fetal heart rate tracings contain any of the following.
  - ▸ Baseline rate
    - ▹ Tachycardia
    - ▹ Bradycardia not accompanied by absent baseline variability
  - ▸ Baseline FHR variability
    - ▹ Minimal baseline variability
    - ▹ Absent baseline variability not accompanied by recurrent decelerations
    - ▹ Marked baseline variability
  - ▸ Episodic or periodic decelerations
    - ▹ Prolonged fetal heart rate deceleration greater than 2 min but less than 10 min
    - ▹ Recurrent late decelerations with moderate baseline variability
    - ▹ Recurrent variable decelerations with minimal or moderate baseline variability
    - ▹ Variable decelerations with additional characteristics, including "overshoots," "shoulders," or slow return to baseline fetal heart rate
  - ▸ Accelerations
    - ▹ Absence of induced accelerations after fetal stimulation
- Category III – Category III fetal heart rate tracings include either:
  - ▸ Sinusoidal pattern
  - ▸ Absent baseline fetal heart rate variability and any of the following
    - ▹ Recurrent variable decelerations
    - ▹ Recurrent late decelerations
    - ▹ Bradycardia
- Each uterine contraction is comprised of the following.
  - Increment – The beginning of the contraction as intensity is increasing.
  - Acme – The peak intensity of the contraction.
  - Decrement – The decline of the contraction intensity as the contraction is ending.
- Nonreassuring FHR patterns are associated with fetal hypoxia and include the following.
  - Fetal bradycardia
  - Fetal tachycardia
  - Absence of FHR variability
  - Late decelerations
  - Variable decelerations

FHR PATTERNS	
CAUSES/COMPLICATIONS	NURSING INTERVENTIONS
Accelerations (variable transitory increase in the FHR above baseline of 15/min lasting 15 seconds or more)	
› Healthy fetal/placental exchange › Intact fetal central nervous system (CNS) response to fetal movement › Vaginal exam › Fundal pressure	› Reassuring › No interventions required › Indicate reactive nonstress test
Fetal bradycardia (FHR less than 110/min for 10 min or more)	
› Uteroplacental insufficiency › Umbilical cord prolapse › Maternal hypotension › Maternal hypoglycemia › Prolonged umbilical cord compression › Fetal congenital heart block › Anesthetic medications	› Discontinue oxytocin (Pitocin) if it is being infused. › Help the client into a side-lying position. › Administer oxygen (8 to 10 L/min by mask). › Assist with the start of an IV line if one is not in place. › Monitor the administration of a tocolytic medication as prescribed. › Notify the provider.
Fetal tachycardia (FHR greater than 160/min for 10 min or more)	
› Maternal infection, chorioamnionitis › Fetal anemia › Fetal heart failure › Fetal cardiac dysrhythmias › Maternal use of cocaine or methamphetamines › Maternal dehydration	› If maternal fever exists, administer antipyretics as prescribed. › Administer oxygen (8 to 10 L/min by mask). › Monitor the administration of bolus IV fluids.
Decrease or loss of FHR variability (decrease or loss of irregular fluctuations in the baseline of the FHR)	
› Medications that depress the CNS, such as narcotics, barbiturates, tranquilizers, or general anesthetics › Fetal hypoxemia with resulting acidosis › Fetal sleep cycle › Congenital abnormalities	› Stimulate the fetal scalp. › Assist provider with application of scalp electrode. › Position the client into a left-lateral position.
Early deceleration of FHR (slowing of FHR with start of contraction with return of FHR to baseline at end of contraction)	
› Compression of the fetal head resulting from uterine contraction › Vaginal exam › Fundal pressure	› No intervention required.

FHR PATTERNS	
CAUSES/COMPLICATIONS	NURSING INTERVENTIONS
Late deceleration of FHR (slowing of FHR after contraction has started with return of FHR to baseline well after contraction has ended)	
› Uteroplacental insufficiency causing inadequate fetal oxygenation › Maternal hypotension, abruptio placentae, uterine hyperstimulation with oxytocin (Pitocin)	› Place the client to a side-lying position. › Assist with the start of an IV line if not in place or increase the IV rate. › Discontinue oxytocin (Pitocin) if being infused. › Administer oxygen 8 to 10 L/min per mask. › Notify the provider. › Prepare for an assisted vaginal birth or cesarean birth.
Variable deceleration of FHR (transitory, abrupt slowing of FHR less than 110 beats/min, variable in duration, intensity, and timing in relation to uterine contraction)	
› Umbilical cord compression › Short cord › Prolapsed cord › Nuchal cord (around fetal neck) › Oligohydramnios	› Change the client's position from side to side or into knee-chest. › Discontinue oxytocin (Pitocin) if it is being infused. › Administer oxygen at 8 to 10 L/min per mask. › Perform or assist with a vaginal examination. › Assist with an amnioinfusion if ordered.

- Nursing Actions
  - Preparation of the client
    - Use Leopold maneuvers to locate the fetal presenting part and the optimal location for placement of the ultrasound transducer for the best possible auscultation of FHR.
    - Palpate uterine activity at the fundus to identify proper placement location for the tocotransducer to monitor uterine contractions.
  - Ongoing care
    - Provide information regarding the procedure to the client and the client's partner during placement and adjustments of the fetal monitor equipment.
    - Encourage frequent maternal position changes. Explain to the client that adjustments of the monitor may be necessary with position changes.
    - If the client needs to void and can ambulate, and it is not contraindicated, the nurse can disconnect the external monitor for the client to use the bathroom.
    - If disconnecting of FHR monitor is contraindicated or internal FHR monitor is being used, the nurse can bring the client a bedpan.

- Description of Procedure
  - Continuous internal fetal monitoring
    - Continuous internal fetal monitoring with a scalp electrode is performed by attaching a small spiral electrode to the presenting part of the fetus to monitor the FHR. The electrode wires are then attached to a leg plate that is placed on the client's thigh and then attached to the fetal monitor.
    - Continuous internal fetal monitoring may be used in conjunction with an intrauterine pressure catheter (IUPC), which is a solid or fluid-filled transducer placed inside the client's uterine cavity to monitor the frequency, duration, and intensity of contractions. The average pressure is usually 50 to 85 mm Hg.
      - Advantages of internal fetal monitoring
        - ‣ Early detection of abnormal FHR patterns suggestive of fetal distress
        - ‣ Accurate measurement of uterine contraction intensity
        - ‣ Accurate assessment of FHR variability
        - ‣ Allows greater maternal freedom of movement without compromising tracing
      - Disadvantages of internal fetal monitoring
        - ‣ Membranes must have ruptured to use internal monitoring
        - ‣ Cervix must be adequately dilated to a minimum of 2 to 3 cm
        - ‣ Presenting part must have descended enough to place electrode
        - ‣ Potential risk of injury to fetus if electrode is not properly applied
        - ‣ Contraindicated with vaginal bleeding
        - ‣ Potential risk of infection to the client and the fetus
        - ‣ A provider, nurse practitioner/midwife, or specially trained registered nurse must perform this procedure
- Nursing Actions
  - Preparation of the client
    - Ensure electronic fetal monitoring equipment is functioning properly.
    - Use aseptic techniques if assisting with procedures.
  - Ongoing care
    - Monitor maternal vital signs and obtain maternal temperature every 1 to 2 hr.
    - Encourage frequent repositioning of the client. If the client is lying supine, place a wedge under one of the client's hips to tilt her uterus.
- Complications
  - Misinterpretation of FHR patterns
  - Maternal or fetal infection
  - Fetal trauma if fetal monitoring electrode or IUPC are inserted into the vagina improperly
  - Supine hypotension secondary to internal monitor placement

APPLICATION EXERCISES

1. A nurse is assisting with the care of a client in active labor. Which of the following will Leopold maneuvers assist the nurse in determining? (Select all that apply.)

_____ A. Presenting part

_____ B. Fetal attitude

_____ C. Fetal lie

_____ D. Position of the cervix

_____ E. Degree of fetal descent into the pelvis

2. A nurse is assisting with the care of a client being induced for labor who is being monitored by an external electronic fetal monitor. The nurse notes that the FHR variability is decreased and resembles a straight line. The client has not received any pain medication. Which of the following should occur first before the nurse can apply an internal scalp electrode?

A. Dilation

B. Rupture of membranes

C. Effacement

D. Engagement

3. A newly licensed nurse is reviewing a fetal monitor tracing of a client in active labor with the charge nurse. Which of the following should the nurse recognize as being associated with fetal hypoxia? (Select all that apply.)

_____ A. Fetal bradycardia

_____ B. Fetal tachycardia

_____ C. Absence of FHR variability

_____ D. Early decelerations

_____ E. Variable decelerations

4. A charge nurse is discussing the potential causes of variable decelerations with a newly licensed nurse. Which of the following should she include in the teaching? (Select all that apply.)

_____ A. Short umbilical cord

_____ B. Polyhydramnios

_____ C. Umbilical cord compression

_____ D. Uteroplacental insufficiency

_____ E. Nuchal cord

5. A nurse is assisting with the care of a client who is in labor and observes late decelerations on the electronic fetal monitor. Which of the following is the first action the nurse should take?

A. Assist the client into the left-lateral position.

B. Assist with the application of a fetal scalp electrode.

C. Assist with the insertion of an IV catheter.

D. Assist the nurse with a vaginal exam.

6. A nurse is assisting with the care in labor and delivery, and the charge nurse is reviewing intermittent fetal auscultation and uterine contraction palpation with her. What should be included in the review? Use the ATI Active Learning Template: Therapeutic Procedure to complete this item to include the following:

A. Indications: Describe four situations when this procedure should be performed.

B. Interpretation of Findings: Describe normal expected FHR findings.

C. Nursing Actions:
- Preprocedure: Describe the three types of devices that are used to auscultate FHR.
- Intraprocedure: Identify the time frame for counting FHR to determine the baseline rate and when auscultation should take place.

APPLICATION EXERCISES KEY

1. A. **CORRECT:** Using Leopold maneuvers to palpate the maternal uterus will assist the nurse in determining the presenting part.

    B. **CORRECT:** Using Leopold maneuvers to palpate the maternal uterus will assist the nurse in determining the fetal attitude.

    C. **CORRECT:** Using Leopold maneuvers to palpate the maternal uterus will assist the nurse in determining the fetal lie.

    D. INCORRECT: Using Leopold maneuvers to palpate the maternal uterus will not assist the nurse in determining the position of the cervix.

    E. **CORRECT:** Using Leopold maneuvers to palpate the maternal uterus will assist the nurse in determining the degree of fetal descent into the pelvis.

     NCLEX® Connection: Health Promotion and Maintenance, Ante/Intra/Postpartum and Newborn Care

2. A. INCORRECT: The cervix must be dilated 2 to 3 cm before internal monitoring can be used, but this is not the first criterion to consider.

    B. **CORRECT:** The membranes must be ruptured prior to the insertion of an internal electrode or intrauterine pressure catheter.

    C. INCORRECT: Effacement of the cervix must occur before internal monitoring can be used, but this is not the first criterion to consider.

    D. INCORRECT: Engagement of the presenting part must occur before internal monitoring can be used, but this is not the first criterion to consider.

     NCLEX® Connection: Health Promotion and Maintenance, Ante/Intra/Postpartum and Newborn Care

3. A. **CORRECT:** The nurse should recognize fetal bradycardia as a nonreassuring FHR pattern associated with fetal hypoxia.

    B. **CORRECT:** The nurse should recognize fetal tachycardia as a nonreassuring FHR pattern associated with fetal hypoxia.

    C. **CORRECT:** The nurse should recognize absence of FHR variability as a nonreassuring FHR pattern associated with fetal hypoxia.

    D. INCORRECT: The nurse should recognize early decelerations occur with cervical dilation and descent, but are not associated with fetal hypoxia.

    E. **CORRECT:** The nurse should recognize variable decelerations as a nonreassuring FHR pattern associated with fetal hypoxia.

     NCLEX® Connection: Health Promotion and Maintenance, Ante/Intra/Postpartum and Newborn Care

4.   A. **CORRECT:** A short umbilical cord can cause variable decelerations.

     B. INCORRECT: Oligohydramnios, rather than polyhydramnios, causes variable decelerations.

     C. **CORRECT:** Umbilical cord compression can cause variable decelerations.

     D. INCORRECT: Uteroplacental insufficiency results in late decelerations.

     E. **CORRECT:** A nuchal cord can cause variable decelerations.

     Ⓝ NCLEX® Connection: Health Promotion and Maintenance, Ante/Intra/Postpartum and Newborn Care

5.   A. **CORRECT:** The greatest risk to the fetus during late decelerations is uteroplacental insufficiency. The initial nursing action should be to place the client into the left-lateral position to increase uteroplacental perfusion.

     B. INCORRECT: The application of a fetal scalp electrode will assist in the assessment of fetal well-being, but this is not the first action the nurse should take.

     C. INCORRECT: Inserting an IV catheter is an intervention for late decelerations, but this is not the first action the nurse should take.

     D. INCORRECT: The nurse can perform a vaginal exam to determine dilation, but this is not the first action the nurse should take.

     Ⓝ NCLEX® Connection: Health Promotion and Maintenance, Ante/Intra/Postpartum and Newborn Care

6.   *Using the ATI Active Learning Template: Therapeutic Procedure*

     A. Indications
        - Rupture of membranes, spontaneously or artificially
        - Preceding and subsequent to ambulation
        - Prior to and following administration of or a change in medication analgesia
        - At the peak action of anesthesia
        - Following vaginal examination
        - Following expulsion of an enema
        - After urinary catheterization
        - In the event of abnormal or excessive uterine contractions

     B. Interpretation of Findings
        - A normal, reassuring FHR is 110 to 160/min with increases and deceases from baseline.

     C. Nursing Actions
        - Preprocedure
           ○ Hand-held Doppler ultrasound
           ○ Ultrasound stethoscope
           ○ Fetoscope
        - Intraprocedure
           ○ Count FHR for 30 to 60 seconds to determine the baseline rate.
           ○ Auscultate during and for 30 seconds following the completion of a contraction.

     Ⓝ NCLEX® Connection: Health Promotion and Maintenance, Ante/Intra/Postpartum and Newborn Care

UNIT 3   Postpartum Nursing Care

CHAPTERS

> Nursing Care of the Client During the Postpartum Period
> Complications of the Postpartum Period

NCLEX® CONNECTIONS

When reviewing the chapters in this unit, keep in mind the relevant sections of the NCLEX® outline, in particular:

Client Needs: Health Promotion and Maintenance

> Relevant topics/tasks include:
  » Ante/Intra/Postpartum and Newborn Care
    > Perform care of postpartum client.
  » Data Collection Techniques
    > Collect baseline physical data.
    > Reinforce client teaching on infant care skills.
    > Monitor recovery of stable postpartum client.
  » Developmental Stages and Transitions
    > Assist client with expected life transition.

Client Needs: Pharmacological Therapies

> Relevant topics/tasks include:
  » Expected Actions/Outcomes
    > Apply knowledge of pathophysiology when addressing client pharmacological agents.

Client Needs: Physiological Adaptations

> Relevant topics/tasks include:
  » Alterations in Body Systems
    > Identify signs and symptoms of an infection.
    > Provide care for a client experiencing complications of pregnancy/labor and/or delivery.

Overview

- The postpartum period, or puerperium, includes physiological and psychosocial adjustments. This period begins at the start of the fourth stage of labor (1 to 4 hr after the delivery of the placenta) and ends when the body returns to the prepregnant state. This process takes approximately 6 weeks.

- The greatest risks during the postpartum period are hemorrhage, shock, and infection.

- Nurses should perform postpartum data collection per facility protocols. Clients who have stable vital signs usually are monitored every 15 min x 4 for the first hour, every 30 min x 2 for the second hr, hourly x 2 for at least 2 hr, then every 4 to 8 hr.

 View Video: Postpartum Data Collection

- Additional data is collected using the acronym BUBBLE.

  - B – Breasts

  - U – Uterus (fundal height, uterine placement, and consistency)

  - B – Bowel and GI function

  - B – Bladder function

  - L – Lochia (color, odor, consistency, and amount [COCA])

  - E – Episiotomy (edema, ecchymosis, approximation)

- Thermoregulation

  - Data collection

    - Postpartum chill, which occurs in the first 2 hr puerperium, is an uncontrollable shaking chill experienced by clients immediately following birth. Postpartum chill is possibly related to a nervous system response, vasomotor changes, a shift in fluids, and/or the work of labor. This is a normal occurrence unless accompanied by an elevated temperature.

  - Nursing actions

    - Provide clients with warm blankets and fluids.

  - Client education

    - Reassure clients that these chills are a self-limiting common occurrence that will only last a short while.

- Fundus
  - Data collection
    - Physical changes of the uterus include involution of the uterus. Involution occurs with contractions of the uterine smooth muscle, whereby the uterus returns to its prepregnant state. The uterus also rapidly decreases in size from approximately 1,000 g (2.2 lb) to 50 to 60 g (less than 2 oz) over 6 weeks with the fundal height steadily descending into the pelvis approximately one fingerbreadth (1 cm) per day.
    - Immediately after delivery, the fundus should be firm, midline with the umbilicus, and approximately at the level of the umbilicus. At 12 hr postpartum, the fundus can be palpated at 1 cm above the umbilicus.
    - Every 24 hr, the fundus should descend approximately 1 to 2 cm. It should be halfway between the symphysis pubis and the umbilicus by the sixth postpartum day.

 View Image: Fundal Height

    - By day 10, the uterus should lie within the true pelvis and should not be palpable.
  - Nursing actions
    - Explain the procedure to the client.
    - Apply clean gloves, and place a lower perineal pad under the client's buttocks.
    - Cup one hand just above the symphysis pubis to support the lower segment of the uterus. With the other hand, palpate the client's abdomen to locate the fundus.
      - Determine the fundal height by placing fingers on the abdomen and measuring how many fingerbreadths (centimeters) fit between the fundus and the umbilicus above, below, or at the umbilical level.
      - Determine if the fundus is midline in the pelvis or displaced laterally (caused by a full bladder).
      - Determine if the fundus is firm or boggy. If the fundus is boggy (not firm), lightly massage the fundus in a circular motion.
      - Observe lochia flow as the fundus is palpated.
    - Document the fundal height, location, and uterine consistency.
    - Monitor clients receiving oxytocics (oxytocin [Pitocin], methylergonovine maleate [Methergine], and carboprost tromethamine [Hemabate]) to promote uterine contractions and to prevent hemorrhage.

    - Monitor for hypotension with oxytocin administration.
    - Monitor for hypertension with administration of methylergonovine maleate, ergonovine maleate, and carboprost tromethamine.
  - Client education
    - Encourage early breastfeeding for clients who are lactating. This will stimulate the production of natural oxytocin and help prevent hemorrhage.
    - Encourage frequent emptying of the bladder every 2 to 3 hr to prevent uterine displacement and atony.

- Lochia
  - Data collection
    - Three stages of lochia (vaginal discharge)
      - Lochia rubra – Bright red color, bloody consistency, fleshy odor, possible small clots, transient flow increases during breastfeeding and upon rising. Lasts 1 to 3 days after delivery.
      - Lochia serosa – Pinkish brown color and serosanguineous consistency. Lasts from approximately day 4 to day 10 after delivery.
      - Lochia alba – Yellowish, white creamy color, fleshy odor. Lasts from approximately day 11 beyond 6 weeks postpartum.
    - Lochia amount is determined by the quantity of saturation on the perineal pad.
      - Scant (less than 2.5 cm)
      - Light (less than 10 cm)
      - Moderate (greater than 10 cm)
      - Heavy (one pad saturated within 2 hr)
      - Excessive blood loss (one pad saturated in 15 min or less or pooling of blood under buttocks)

 View Image: Vaginal Bleeding

    - Monitor the lochia flow for normal color, amount, and consistency.
      - Expected findings
        - Lochia typically trickles from the vaginal opening, but flows more steadily during uterine contractions.
        - A gush of lochia with the expression of clots and dark blood that has pooled in the vagina can occur with ambulation or massage of the uterus.
      - Abnormal findings
        - Excessive spurting of bright red blood from the vagina, possibly indicating a cervical or vaginal tear
        - Numerous large clots and excessive blood loss (saturation of one pad in 15 min or less), which can be indicative of a hemorrhage
        - Foul odor, which is suggestive of an infection
        - Persistent lochia rubra in the early postpartum period beyond day three, which can indicate retained placental fragments
        - Continued flow of lochia serosa or alba beyond the normal length of time can indicate endometritis, especially if it is accompanied by a fever, pain, or abdominal tenderness
  - Nursing actions
    - Notify the provider.
    - Administer antibiotics if indicated.
    - Assist with emergency care of clients.
  - Client education
    - Instruct the client to notify the provider of abnormal findings of lochia.

- Cervix, Vagina, and Perineum
  - Data collection
    - The cervix is soft directly after birth and can be edematous, bruised, and have some small lacerations. Within 2 to 3 days postpartum, it shortens and regains its form, becoming firm with the os gradually closing.
    - The vagina, which has distended, gradually returns to its prepregnancy size with the reappearance of rugae and a thickening of the vaginal mucosa. However, muscle tone is never restored completely.
    - The soft tissues of the perineum can be erythematous and edematous, especially in areas of an episiotomy or lacerations. Hematomas or hemorrhoids can be present. The pelvic floor muscles can be overstretched and weak.
    - Monitor for cervical, vaginal, and perineal healing.
    - Observe for perineal erythema, edema, and hematoma.
    - Check episiotomy and lacerations for approximation, drainage, quantity, and quality.
      - A bright red trickle of blood from the episiotomy site in the early postpartum period is a normal finding.
  - Nursing actions
    - Encourage clients to eat a well-balanced diet, with adequate fruits, vegetables, fiber, and fluids.
    - Instruct clients about proper cleansing to prevent infection. Tell clients to:
      - Wash hands thoroughly before and after voiding.
      - Use a squeeze bottle filled with warm water or antiseptic solution after each voiding to cleanse the perineal area.
      - Clean the perineal area from front to back (urethra to anus).
      - Blot dry. Do not wipe.
      - Use a topical application of antiseptic cream or spray.
      - Change the perineal pad from front to back after voiding or defecating.
    - Promote comfort measures.
      - Apply ice packs to the client's perineum for the first 24 to 48 hr to reduce edema and provide anesthetic effect.
      - Encourage sitz baths at 40° C (104° F) or cooler at least twice a day.
      - Administer analgesia, such as nonopioids (acetaminophen [Tylenol]), nonsteroidal anti-inflammatories (ibuprofen [Advil]), and opioids (codeine, hydrocodone) for pain and discomfort.
      - Apply topical anesthetics (Americaine spray or Dermoplast) to the client's perineal area as needed or witch hazel compresses (Tuck's) to the rectal area for hemorrhoids.

Ⓠ
PCC

- ○ Client education
    - ▪ Recommend clients to avoid sexual intercourse until the episiotomy/laceration is healed, vaginal discharge has turned white (lochia alba), and a provider has verbalized that sexual intercourse can resume. This usually takes 2 to 4 weeks, but can be longer, depending on the patient. Over-the-counter lubricants can be needed during the first 6 weeks due to a decrease in estrogen that reduces vaginal lubrication.
    - ▪ Inform clients that physiological reactions to sexual activity can be slower and less intense for the first 3 months following birth.
    - ▪ Advise clients to begin using contraception upon resumption of sexual activity and that pregnancy can occur while breastfeeding even though menses has not returned.
    - ▪ Inform clients who are breastfeeding that menses might not resume for 3 months or until cessation of breastfeeding.
    - ▪ Inform clients who are not breastfeeding that menses might not resume until around 4 to 10 weeks.

- Breasts
    - ○ Data collection
        - ▪ Secretion of colostrum occurs during pregnancy and 2 to 3 days immediately after birth. Milk is produced 2 to 3 days after the delivery of the newborn.
        - ▪ Monitor clients for:
            - ▫ Redness and tenderness of the breast.
            - ▫ Cracked nipples and indications of mastitis (infection in a milk duct of the breast with concurrent flu-like symptoms).
    - ○ Nursing actions
        - ▪ Encourage early-demand breastfeeding, which also stimulates the production of natural oxytocin and helps prevent uterine hemorrhage.
        - ▪ Assist the client too a comfortable position and have her try various positions during breastfeeding (cradle hold, side-lying, and football hold). Explain how varying positions can prevent nipple soreness.
        - ▪ Reinforce to clients the importance of proper latch techniques (the newborn takes in part of the areola and nipple, not just the tip of the nipple) to prevent nipple soreness.
    - ○ Client education
        - ▪ Instruct clients to wear a well-fitting bra continuously for the first 72 hr after birth.
        - ▪ For clients who are lactating
            - ▫ Emphasize the importance of hand hygiene prior to breastfeeding to prevent infection.
            - ▫ Instruct clients to:
                - ▸ Completely empty the breasts at each feeding. Massaging the breasts during feeding can help with emptying.
                - ▸ Allow newborns to nurse on demand. Allow newborns to feed 15 to 20 min per breast or until the breast softens. Begin the next breastfeeding session on the breast that was not completely emptied.

    □ Instruct clients to manage breast engorgement.

    □ Apply cool compresses between feedings.

    □ Apply warm compresses or take a warm shower prior to breastfeeding.

    □ Apply cold cabbage to the breasts to decrease swelling and relieve discomfort. However, frequent application of cabbage leaves can decrease milk supply.

    □ Instruct clients who have flat nipples to roll the nipples between her fingers just before breastfeeding to help them become more erect and make it easier for newborns to latch on.

    □ Instruct clients who have sore nipples to apply a small amount of breast milk to the nipples and allow it to air-dry after breastfeeding.

    □ Instruct clients to apply breast creams as prescribed and wear breast shields in their bra to soften the nipples if they are irritated and cracked.

    □ Encourage clients to drink enough fluids to satisfy thirst.

    □ The ideal diet for the lactating mother is well balanced, consisting of nutrient-dense foods. Most women achieve this by adding 300 to 500 calories per day to their diet.

- For nonlactating women

    □ Instruct clients to avoid breast stimulation and running warm water over the breasts for prolonged periods until no longer lactating.

    □ Instruct clients to manage breast engorgement, which can occur on the third or fifth postpartum day.

    □ Instruct clients to apply cold compresses, 15 min on and 45 min off.

    □ Instruct clients to place fresh cabbage leaves inside the bra.

    □ Instruct clients to take a mild analgesic for pain and discomfort.

- Cardiovascular System and Fluid and Hematologic Status

    ○ Data collection

        ■ The cardiovascular system undergoes a decrease in blood volume during the postpartum period related to:

            □ Blood loss during childbirth (average is 500 mL in an uncomplicated vaginal delivery and 1,000 mL for a cesarean birth).

            □ Diaphoresis and diuresis of the excess fluid accumulated during the last part of the pregnancy. Loss occurs within the first 2 to 3 days postdelivery.

        ■ Increased Hct and Hgb values are present immediately after delivery for up to 72 hr. Leukocytosis (white blood cell count elevation) of up to 25,000/mm^3 occurs for the first 10 to 14 days without the presence of infection and then returns to normal.

        ■ Coagulation factors and fibrinogen levels increase during pregnancy and remain elevated for 2 to 3 weeks postpartum. Hypercoagulability predisposes the postpartum woman to thrombus formation and thromboembolism.

        ■ Blood pressure is usually unchanged with an uncomplicated pregnancy, but can have an insignificant slight transient increase.

- Possible orthostatic hypotension within the first 48 hr postpartum can occur immediately after standing up with feelings of faintness or dizziness resulting from splanchnic (viscera/internal organs) engorgement that can occur after birth.

- Elevation of pulse, stroke volume, and cardiac output for the first hour postpartum occurs and then gradually decreases to a prepregnant state baseline by 8 to 10 weeks.

- Elevation of temperature to 38° C (100° F) resulting from dehydration after labor during the first 24 hr can occur, but should return to normal after 24 hr postpartum.

- ○ Nursing actions

  - Monitor vital signs per facility protocol.

  - Inspect legs for redness, swelling, and warmth, which are signs of venous thrombosis.

  - Encourage early ambulation to prevent venous stasis and thrombosis.

  - Apply antiembolism hose to the lower extremities of clients who are at high-risk for developing venous stasis and thrombosis. The hose should be removed as soon as clients are ambulating.

  - Administer medications as prescribed.

- Gastrointestinal System and Bowel Function

  - ○ Data collection

    - An increased appetite following delivery

    - Constipation with bowel evacuation delayed until 2 to 3 days after birth

    - Hemorrhoids

  - ○ Nursing actions

    - Monitor for reports of hunger.

    - Check for bowel sounds and the return of normal bowel function.

      - □ Spontaneous bowel movement might not occur for 2 to 3 days after delivery secondary to decreased intestinal muscle tone during labor and puerperium and prelabor diarrhea and dehydration. Clients can anticipate discomfort with defecation because of perineal tenderness, episiotomy, lacerations, or hemorrhoids.

    - Observe the rectal area for varicosities (hemorrhoids).

    - Administer stool softeners (docusate sodium) to prevent constipation.

  - ○ Client education

    - Encourage clients to eat a well-balanced diet, with adequate fruits, vegetables, high-fiber food sources, and fluids.

    - Encourage clients to ambulate.

- Urinary System and Bladder Function

  - ○ Data collection

    - Urinary retention secondary to loss of bladder elasticity and tone and/or loss of bladder sensation resulting from trauma, medications, or anesthesia.

    - A distended bladder as a result of urinary retention can cause uterine atony and displacement to one side, usually to the right. The ability of the uterus to contract is also lessened.

    - Postpartal diuresis with increased urinary output begins within 12 hr of delivery.

- ○ Nursing actions
  - ▪ Determine the client's ability to void every 2 to 3 hr (perineal/urethral edema can cause pain and difficulty in voiding during the first 24 to 48 hr).
  - ▪ Observe the client's bladder elimination pattern (client should void every 2 to 3 hr).
  - ▪ Monitor for manifestations of a distended bladder
    - □ Fundal height above the umbilicus or baseline level
    - □ Fundus displaced from the midline over to the side
    - □ Bladder bulges above the symphysis pubis
    - □ Excessive lochia
    - □ Tenderness over the bladder area
    - □ Frequent voiding of less than 150 mL of urine is indicative of urinary retention with overflow
  - ▪ Insert a straight or indwelling urinary catheter for bladder distention if clients are unable to void to ensure complete emptying of the bladder and allow uterine involution.
- ○ Client education
  - ▪ Encourage clients to empty their bladder frequently (every 2 to 3 hr) to prevent possible displacement of the uterus and atony.
- Musculoskeletal System
  - ○ Data collection
    - ▪ By 6 to 8 weeks after birth
      - □ Joints return to their pregnant state and are completely restabilized. Feet can remain permanently increased in size.
      - □ Muscle tone begins to be restored throughout the body with the removal of progesterone's effect following delivery of the placenta.
    - ▪ The rectus abdominis muscles of the abdomen and the pubococcygeal muscle tone are restored following placental expulsion.
  - ○ Nursing actions
    - ▪ Monitor the abdominal wall for diastasis recti (a separation of the rectus muscle) of 2 to 4 cm. It usually resolves within 6 weeks.
  - ○ Client education
    - ▪ Reinforce the importance of postpartum strengthening exercises, advising clients to start with simple exercises, and then gradually progress to more strenuous ones.
    - ▪ Kegel exercises use the same muscles as starting and stopping the flow of urine. Have clients relax and contract the pelvic floor muscles 10 times, eight times a day.
    - ▪ Pelvic tilt exercises strengthen back muscles and relieve strain on the lower back. Instruct clients to alternately arch and straighten the back.
    - ▪ Advise clients to use good body mechanics and proper posture.

- Recommend that clients:
  - Not lift anything heavier than the newborn.
  - Avoid sitting for prolonged periods of time with legs crossed (to prevent thrombophlebitis).
  - Limit stair-climbing for the first few weeks postpartum.
  - To not drive for the first 2 weeks postpartum, or while taking opioids for pain control.
- Advise clients who have had a cesarean birth to:
  - Postpone abdominal exercises until about 4 weeks after delivery, or as directed by the provider.
  - Wait until the 6-week follow-up visit before performing strenuous exercise, heavy lifting, or excessive stair-climbing.

- Immune System
  - Nursing actions
    - Review rubella status – A client who has a titer of less than 1:8 is administered a subcutaneous injection of rubella vaccine or a measles, mumps and rubella vaccine during the postpartum period to protect a subsequent fetus from malformations. Clients should not get pregnant for 1 month following the immunization.
    - Review hepatitis B status – Newborns born to infected mothers should receive the hepatitis B vaccine and the hepatitis B immune globulin within 12 hr of birth.
    - Review Rh status – All Rh-negative mothers who have newborns, and are Rh-positive, must be given $RH_o(D)$ immune globulin (RhoGAM) IM within 72 hr of the newborn being born to suppress antibody formation in the mother.
    - Review varicella status – If the client has no immunity, varicella vaccine is administered before discharge. The client should not get pregnant for 1 month following the immunization. A second dose of vaccine is given at 4 to 8 weeks.
    - Review tetanus diphtheria acellular pertussis vaccine status – The vaccine is recommended for women who have not previously received the vaccine. Administer prior to discharge or as soon as possible in the postpartum period.
  - Client education
    - Remind clients who receive both the rubella vaccine and RhoGAM to return to the provider after 3 months to determine if immunity to rubella has developed.

- Comfort and Rest
  - Nursing actions
    - Monitor pain related to episiotomy, lacerations, incisions, afterpains, and sore nipples.
    - Determine location, type, and quality of the pain to guide nursing interventions and client instruction.
    - Administer pain medications as prescribed.

- Maternal Adaptation
  - Data collection
    - Psychosocial adaptation and maternal adjustment begin during pregnancy as clients go through commitment, attachment, and preparation for the birth of the newborn. During the first 2 to 6 weeks after birth, clients go through a period of acquaintance with her newborn, as well as physical restoration. During this time she also focuses on competently caring for her newborn. Finally, the act of achieving maternal identity is accomplished around 4 months following birth. It is important to note that these stages can overlap, and are variable based on maternal, newborn, and environmental factors.
    - Phases of maternal role attainment
      - Dependent: taking-in phase
        - First 24 to 48 hr
        - Focus is on meeting personal needs
        - Rely on others for assistance
        - Excited, talkative; need to review birth experience with others
      - Dependent-independent: taking-hold phase
        - Begins on day 2 or 3; up to 10 days to several weeks
        - Focus on baby care and improving care-giving competency
        - Want to take charge but need acceptance from others
        - Want to learn and practice
      - Interdependent: letting-go phase
        - Focus on family as a unit
        - Resumption of role (intimate partner, individual)
    - Monitor clients for behaviors that facilitate and indicate mother-infant bonding.
      - Considers the newborn a family member
      - Holds the newborn face to face (en face) maintaining eye contact
      - Assigns meaning to the newborn's behavior and views positively
      - Identifies the newborn's unique characteristics and relates them to those of other family members
      - Names the infant (indicates that bonding is occurring)
      - Touches the newborn and maintains close physical proximity and contact
      - Provides physical care for the newborn such as feeding and diapering
      - Responds to the newborn's cries
      - Smiles at, talks to, and sings to the newborn
    - Monitor for behaviors that impair and indicate a lack of mother-infant bonding.
      - Apathy when the newborn cries
      - Disgust when the newborn voids, stools, or spits up
      - Expression of disappointment in the newborn

◻ Turning away from the newborn

◻ Not seeking close physical proximity to the newborn

◻ Not talking about the newborn's unique features

◻ Handling the newborn roughly

◻ Ignoring the newborn entirely

■ Monitor for indications of mood swings, conflict about maternal role, and personal insecurity.

◻ Feelings of being "down"

◻ Feelings of inadequacy

◻ Feelings of anxiety related to ineffective breastfeeding

◻ Emotional lability with frequent crying

◻ Flat affect and being withdrawn

◻ Feeling unable to care for the newborn

○ Nursing actions

■ Provide a quiet and private environment that enhances the family bonding process.

■ Facilitate the bonding process by placing the newborn skin-to-skin with the mother soon after birth in an en face position.

■ Encourage parents to bond with their newborn through cuddling, feeding, diapering, and inspection.

○ Client education

■ Provide frequent praise, support, and reassurance to the mother as she moves toward independence in caring for her newborn and adjusting to her maternal role.

■ Encourage parents to express their feelings, fears, and anxieties about caring for their newborn.

• Paternal Adaptation

○ Data collection

■ Paternal transition to fatherhood consists of a predictable three-stage process during the first few weeks of transition.

◻ Expectations – The father has preconceived ideas about what it will be like to be a father.

◻ Reality – The father discovers that his expectations might not be met. Commonly expressed emotions include feeling sad, frustrated, and jealous. He embraces the need to be actively involved in parenting.

◻ Transition to mastery – The father decides to become actively involved in the care of the newborn.

■ The development of the father-infant bond consists of three stages.

◻ Making a commitment – The father takes the responsibility of parenting.

◻ Becoming connected – The father experiences feelings of attachment to the newborn.

◻ Making room for the newborn – The father modifies his life to include the care of the newborn.

- ○ Nursing actions
  - ▪ Monitor fathers for behaviors that facilitate and indicate father-infant bonding.
    - ▫ Fathers touch, hold, and maintain eye-to-eye contact with their newborn.
    - ▫ Fathers observe newborns for features similar to their own to validate claim of the infant.
    - ▫ Fathers talk, read, and sing to the infant.
  - ▪ Provide education about newborn care when fathers are present.
- ○ Client education
  - ▪ Assist fathers in their transition to fatherhood by providing guidance and involving them as full partners rather than just helpers.
  - ▪ Provide education about infant care when fathers are present, and encourage the father to take a hands-on approach.
  - ▪ Encourage couples to verbalize their concerns and expectations related to newborn care.

- • Sibling Adaptation
  - ○ Data collection
    - ▪ Monitor for positive responses from the sibling.
      - ▫ Interest and concern for the newborn
      - ▫ Increased independence
    - ▪ Monitor for adverse responses from the sibling.
      - ▫ Indications of sibling rivalry and jealousy
      - ▫ Regression in toileting and sleep habits
      - ▫ Aggression toward the newborn
      - ▫ Increased attention-seeking behaviors and whining
  - ○ Nursing actions
    - ▪ Take siblings on a tour of the obstetric unit.
    - ▪ Encourage the parents to:
      - ▫ Let siblings be some of the first to see the newborn.
      - ▫ Provide a gift from the newborn to give the sibling.
      - ▫ Arrange for one parent to spend time with siblings while the other parent is caring for the newborn.
      - ▫ Allow older siblings to help in providing care for the newborn.
      - ▫ Provide toddlers and preschoolers with a doll to care for.

- Family Adaptation
  - Nursing actions
    - Emphasize verbal and nonverbal communication skills between the mother, caregivers, and the infant.
    - Encourage continued support of grandparents and other family members.
    - Provide information regarding community resources for families who have young children.
    - Encourage attendance at parenting classes or support group for new parents. Give the parents information about social networks that provide a support system where they can seek assistance.
- Postpartum Discharge
  - Nursing actions
    - Schedule a postpartum follow-up visit. Following a vaginal delivery, the follow-up visit should take place in 6 weeks. Following a cesarean birth, the visit should take place in 2 weeks.
    - Provide written postpartum and newborn instructions.
    - Instruct clients to report danger signs to the provider.
      - Chills or fever greater than 38° C (100.4° F) for 2 or more days
      - Change in vaginal discharge with increased amount, large clots, and change to a previous lochia color, such as bright red bleeding and a foul odor
      - Episiotomy, laceration, or incision pain that does not resolve with analgesics
      - Foul-smelling drainage, redness, or edema
      - Pain or tenderness in the abdominal or pelvic areas that does not resolve with analgesics
      - Breast(s) with localized areas of pain and tenderness with redness and swelling and/or nipples with cracks or fissures
      - Calves with localized pain and tenderness, redness, and swelling; a lower extremity with either areas of redness and warmth or coolness and paleness
      - Urination with burning, pain, frequency, urgency; urine that is cloudy or has blood
      - Feelings of apathy toward the newborn, inability to provide self- or newborn-care, or feelings that can result in self- or newborn injury

APPLICATION EXERCISES

1. After delivery, the uterus contracts and gradually returns to its prepregnant state. This is referred to as which of the following?

    A. Uterine inversion

    B. Uterine subinvolution

    C. Uterine involution

    D. Uterine exfoliation

2. A nurse is collecting data from a postpartum client. Which of the following findings indicate bladder distension? (Select all that apply.)

    _____ A. Displaced fundus from midline

    _____ B. Excessive lochia

    _____ C. Bladder tenderness

    _____ D. Fundal height below the umbilicus

    _____ E. Bulging bladder above the symphysis pubis

3. A nurse is caring for a family who has a newborn. The father appears very anxious and nervous when the mother asks him to bring her the newborn. Which of the following is an appropriate nursing intervention to promote father-infant bonding?

    A. Hand the father the newborn and insist he change the diaper.

    B. Ask the father why he is so anxious and nervous.

    C. Tell the father that he will get used to the newborn in time.

    D. Provide education about newborn care when the father is present.

4. A nurse in a provider's office is caring for a client who is breastfeeding and is 4 days postpartum. The client reports breast engorgement. Which of the following recommendations should the nurse make?

    A. Apply cold cabbage leaves between feedings.

    B. Place warm compresses right after feedings.

    C. Apply breast milk to the nipples and allow them to air dry.

    D. Use the various newborn positions for feedings.

5. A nurse is reinforcing discharge instructions for a client. Which of the following should the nurse instruct the client to report to the provider?

    A. White vaginal discharge

    B. Cramping during breastfeeding

    C. Sore nipple with cracks and fissures

    D. Decreased response with sexual activity

6. A nurse on a postpartum unit is leading a discussion with a group of clients about perineal care after delivery. What should be included in the discussion? Use the ATI Active Learning Template: Basic Concept to complete this item to include the following sections:

    A. Underlying Principles: Describe three concepts that are the basis for perineal hygiene.

    B. Nursing Interventions:
        • Describe four actions the client should take to prevent infection.
        • Describe four actions the nurse can take to promote client comfort.

APPLICATION EXERCISES KEY

1. A. INCORRECT: Uterine inversion is a condition in which the uterus turns inside out and can be caused by the placenta being removed too vigorously prior to its natural detachment process.

   B. INCORRECT: Uterine subinvolution is the delay of the uterus in returning to the prepregnancy state.

   C. **CORRECT:** Uterine involution is the return of the uterus to the prepregnant state. Postpartum contractions aid in uterine involution.

   D. INCORRECT: Uterine exfoliation is the shedding of the decidua tissue layers.

    NCLEX® Connection: Health Promotion and Maintenance, Ante/Intra/Postpartum and Newborn Care

2. A. **CORRECT:** A distended bladder can cause uterine atony and lateral displacement from the midline, usually to the right.

   B. **CORRECT:** Excessive lochia rubra is a finding associated with bladder distension.

   C. **CORRECT:** Bladder tenderness is a finding associated with bladder distension.

   D. INCORRECT: The fundal height would be above the umbilicus in a client with bladder distension.

   E. **CORRECT:** A bulging bladder above the symphysis pubis is a finding associated with bladder distension.

    NCLEX® Connection: Health Promotion and Maintenance, Ante/Intra/Postpartum and Newborn Care

3. A. INCORRECT: It is not helpful to push the father into infant care activities without first providing education.

   B. INCORRECT: This is a nontherapeutic statement and presumes the nurse knows what the father is feeling.

   C. INCORRECT: This is a nontherapeutic statement and offers the nurse's opinion.

   D. **CORRECT:** Nursing interventions to promote paternal bonding include providing education about infant care and encouraging the father to take a hands-on approach.

   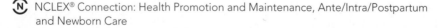 NCLEX® Connection: Health Promotion and Maintenance, Ante/Intra/Postpartum and Newborn Care

4. A. **CORRECT:** The nurse should instruct the client to apply cold cabbage leaves to the breasts between feedings to help with breast engorgement.

    B. INCORRECT: The nurse should instruct the client to apply warm compresses prior to feedings, not immediately after, to assist with the letdown reflex and milk flow.

    C. INCORRECT: The nurse should instruct the client to apply breast milk and to air dry the nipples to help prevent nipple soreness, but this has no effect on breast engorgement.

    D. INCORRECT: The nurse should instruct the client to use various positions for feedings to help prevent nipple soreness, but this has no effect on breast engorgement.

    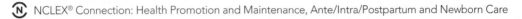 NCLEX® Connection: Health Promotion and Maintenance, Ante/Intra/Postpartum and Newborn Care

5. A. INCORRECT: The nurse should instruct the client that lochia alba, a white vaginal discharge, is an expected finding from 11 days postpartum to approximately 6 weeks following birth.

    B. INCORRECT: The nurse should instruct the client that oxytocin, which is released with breastfeeding, causes the uterus to contract and can cause discomfort.

    C. **CORRECT:** The nurse should instruct the client that a sore nipple that has cracks and fissures is an indication of mastitis and needs to be reported to the provider.

    D. INCORRECT: The nurse should instruct the client that physiological reactions to sexual activity can be slower and less intense for the first 3 months following birth.

    (N) NCLEX® Connection: Health Promotion and Maintenance, Ante/Intra/Postpartum and Newborn Care

6. *Using the ATI Active Learning Template: Basic Concept*

    A. Underlying Principles
    - Promote stool softening.
    - Promote comfort.

    B. Nursing Interventions
    - Prevent infection.
    - Wash hands thoroughly before and after voiding.
    - Use a squeeze bottle with warm water or antiseptic solution after each voiding.
    - Clean the perineal area from front to back.
    - Blot dry. Do not wipe.
    - Use topical application of antiseptic cream or spray sparingly.
    - Change perineal pad from front to back after voiding and defecating.
    - Promote comfort.
    - Apply ice packs to the perineum for 24 to 48 hr.
    - Encourage sitz baths at least twice a day.
    - Administer analgesics.
    - Assist with administering PCA pump after cesarean birth.
    - Apply topical anesthetics to perineal area or witch hazel compresses to the rectal area.

    (N) NCLEX® Connection: Health Promotion and Maintenance, Ante/Intra/Postpartum and Newborn Care

chapter 13 ✈

Overview

- Postpartum complications are unexpected events or occurrences that can happen during the postpartum period. It is imperative for a nurse to have a thorough understanding of each disorder and initiate appropriate nursing interventions to achieve positive outcomes. They include:

    ○ Superficial and deep-vein thrombosis, pulmonary embolus, coagulopathies (idiopathic thrombocytopenic purpura and disseminated intravascular coagulation), postpartum hemorrhage, lacerations and/or hematomas, and postpartum depression.

DEEP-VEIN THROMBOSIS

Overview

- Thrombophlebitis refers to a thrombus that is associated with inflammation.

- Thrombophlebitis of the lower extremities can be of superficial veins or of the deep veins, which are most often of the femoral, saphenous, or popliteal veins.

    ○ Postpartum clients are at risk for a deep-vein thrombosis (DVT) that can lead to a pulmonary embolism.

Data Collection

- Risk Factors

    ○ Pregnancy

    ○ Immobility

    ○ Obesity

    ○ Smoking

    ○ Cesarean birth

    ○ Multiparity

    ○ Greater than 35 years of age

    ○ Previous thromboembolism

- Subjective Data

    ○ Leg pain

    ○ Tenderness

- Objective Data
  - Data collection findings
    - Unilateral swelling, warmth, and redness
    - Warm extremity
    - Calf tenderness
- Diagnostic Procedures
  - Noninvasive method
    - Doppler ultrasound scanning

Patient-Centered Care

- Nursing Care
  - Prevention of thrombophlebitis
    - Initiate early and frequent ambulation during the postpartum period.
    - Instruct clients to avoid prolonged periods of standing, sitting, or immobility.
    - Tell clients to elevate their legs when sitting and to avoid crossing their legs, which will reduce the circulation and exacerbate venous stasis.
    - Recommend for clients to maintain fluid intake of 2 to 3 L of water each day from food and beverage sources to prevent dehydration, which causes circulation to be sluggish.
    - Tell the client to discontinue smoking, which is a known risk factor.
    - Measure the client's lower extremities for fitted elastic thromboembolic hose to lower extremities. Provide thigh-high antiembolism stockings for the client at high risk for venous insufficiency.
  - Management of thrombophlebitis
    - Encourage clients to rest.
    - Facilitate bed rest and elevation of the client's extremity above the level of the heart. (Avoid using a knee gatch or pillow under knees.)
    - Administer intermittent or continuous warm moist compresses.
    - Do NOT massage the affected limb to prevent thrombus from dislodging and becoming an embolus.
    - Monitor the client's leg circumferences.
    - Administer analgesics (nonsteroidal anti-inflammatory agents).
    - Administer anticoagulants for DVT.
- Medications
  - Heparin
    - Anticoagulant
    - Monitor clients receiving IV heparin to prevent formation of other clots and to prevent enlargement of the existing clot.

- Nursing considerations
  - Monitor clients receiving heparin by continuous IV infusion.
  - Ensure protamine sulfate is available to counteract excessive anticoagulation.
  - Monitor aPTT.
- Client education
  - Reinforce teaching with clients to report bleeding from the gums or nose, increased vaginal bleeding, blood in the urine, and frequent bruising.
- Warfarin (Coumadin)
  - Anticoagulant
  - Warfarin is used to prevent the formation of blood clots. It is administered orally and is continued by clients for approximately 3 months.
  - Nursing considerations
    - Phytonadione (vitamin K), the warfarin antidote, should be readily available for prolonged clotting times.
    - Monitor prothrombin time (PT) and INR.
  - Client education
    - Explain to clients to watch for bleeding from the gums or nose, increased vaginal bleeding, blood in the urine, and frequent bruising.
- Enoxaparin (Lovenox)
  - Low molecular weight heparin (LMWH)
  - Lovenox is given subcutaneously to treat or prevent the formation of clots.
  - Nursing considerations
    - Enoxaparin (Lovenox) is given subcutaneously every 12 hr.
    - Routine monitoring of coagulation parameters is not required.
  - Client education
    - Instruct clients to report bleeding from the gums or nose, increased vaginal bleeding, return to lochia rubra after progressing to serosa or alba, blood in the urine, and frequent bruising.
- Care After Discharge
  - Client education
    - Reinforce teaching with clients.
      - Avoid taking aspirin or ibuprofen (increases bleeding tendencies).
      - Use an electric razor for shaving.
      - Avoid alcohol use (inhibits warfarin). If taking warfarin, use a reliable method of contraception (teratogenic) because oral contraceptives are contraindicated due to increased risk for thrombosis.
      - Brush teeth using a soft toothbrush.
      - Avoid rubbing or massaging legs.
      - Avoid periods of prolonged sitting or crossing legs.

- Complications
  - Pulmonary embolus
    - A pulmonary embolus occurs when fragments or an entire clot dislodges, moves into the circulation and enters the pulmonary artery or one of its branches and lodges in a lung, occluding the vessel and obstructing blood flow.
    - Nursing considerations
      - Subjective Data
        - Apprehension
        - Pleuritic chest pain
      - Objective Data
        - Dyspnea
        - Tachypnea
        - Hemoptysis
        - Heart murmurs
        - Peripheral edema
        - Distended neck veins
        - Elevated temperature
        - Hypotension
        - Hypoxia
      - Nursing Care
        - Monitor clients for chills, apprehension, pleuritic chest pain, dyspnea, and tachypnea.
        - Assist with emergency care of the client.
        - Place clients in a semi-Fowler's position with the head of the bed elevated to facilitate breathing.
        - Administer oxygen to clients by mask.
        - Monitor clients receiving thrombolytic therapy.

COAGULOPATHIES (IDIOPATHIC THROMBOCYTOPENIC PURPURA AND DISSEMINATED INTRAVASCULAR COAGULATION)

Overview

- Idiopathic thrombocytopenic purpura (ITP) is a coagulopathy that is an autoimmune disorder in which the life span of platelets is decreased by antiplatelet antibodies. This can result in severe hemorrhage following a cesarean birth or cervical or vaginal lacerations.
- Disseminated intravascular coagulation (DIC) is a coagulopathy in which clotting and anticlotting mechanisms occur at the same time.
- Clients are at risk for both internal and external bleeding as well as damage to organs resulting from ischemia caused by microclots.
- Coagulopathies are suspected when the usual measures to stimulate uterine contractions fail to stop vaginal bleeding.

Data Collection

- Risk Factors
  - Risk factors for ITP are genetic factors inherited from parents.
  - Risk factors for DIC occur secondary to other complications.
    - Abruptio placenta
    - Amniotic fluid embolism
    - HELLP syndrome
    - Fetal death in utero (fetus has died but is retained in the uterus for at least 6 weeks)
    - Severe preeclampsia
    - Septicemia
    - Cardiopulmonary arrest
    - Hemorrhage
    - Hydatidiform mole
- Objective Data
  - Data collection findings
    - Unusual spontaneous bleeding from the client's gums and nose (epistaxis)
    - Oozing, trickling, or flow of blood from incision, lacerations, or episiotomy
    - Petechiae and ecchymoses
    - Excessive bleeding from venipuncture, injection sites, or urinary catheter insertion site
    - Tachycardia and diaphoresis
    - Hematuria
- Laboratory Tests
  - CBC with differential
  - Blood typing and crossmatch
  - Clotting factors
    - Platelet levels (decreased)
    - Fibrinogen levels (decreased)
    - PT (increased)
    - Fibrin split product levels (increased)

Patient-Centered Care

- Nursing Care
  - Monitor clients for bleeding.
  - Monitor urinary output with indwelling urinary catheter.
  - Provide supplemental oxygen.
  - Monitor clients receiving IV fluid replacement and blood and blood products.
  - Monitor laboratory work.

UTERINE ATONY

Overview

- Uterine atony results from the inability of the uterine muscle to contract adequately after birth. This can lead to postpartum hemorrhage.

- Risk Factors

  - Retained placental fragments

  - Prolonged labor

  - Oxytocin (Pitocin) induction or augmentation of labor

  - Overdistention of the uterine muscle (multiparity, multifetal gestations, hydramnios, macrosomic fetus)

  - Precipitous labor

  - Magnesium sulfate administration as a tocolytic

  - Halogenated anesthesia administration

  - Traumatic birth

Data Collection

- Subjective Data

  - Increased vaginal bleeding

- Objective Data

  - Data collection findings

    - A uterus that is larger than normal and boggy with possible lateral displacement on palpation

    - Prolonged lochial discharge

    - Irregular or excessive bleeding

    - Tachycardia and hypotension

    - Skin that is pale, cool, and clammy with poor turgor and pale mucous membranes

  - Diagnostic procedures

    - Bimanual compression or manual exploration of the uterine cavity for retained placental fragments by the primary care provider

    - Surgical management

Patient-Centered Care

- Nursing Care
  - ○ Ensure that the client's urinary bladder is empty.
  - ○ Monitor the following.
    - ▪ Fundal height, consistency, and location
    - ▪ Lochia for quantity, color, and consistency
  - ○ Perform fundal massage if indicated.
    - ▪ If the uterus becomes firm, continue monitoring maternal hemodynamic status.
    - ▪ If uterine atony persists, anticipate surgical intervention.
  - ○ Express clots that can have accumulated in the uterus, but only after the uterus is firmly contracted.
    - ▪ It is critical not to express clots prior to the uterus becoming firmly contracted because pushing on an uncontracted uterus can invert the uterus and result in extensive hemorrhage.
  - ○ Monitor vital signs.
  - ○ Monitor clients receiving IV fluids.

POSTPARTUM HEMORRHAGE

Overview

- Postpartum hemorrhage is considered to occur if clients lose more than 500 mL of blood after a vaginal birth or more than 1,000 mL of blood after a cesarean birth. Two complications that can occur following postpartum hemorrhage are hypovolemic shock and anemia.

Data Collection

- Risk Factors
  - ○ Uterine atony
  - ○ Complications during pregnancy (e.g., placenta previa, abruptio placentae)
  - ○ Prolonged labor
  - ○ Administration of magnesium sulfate therapy during labor
  - ○ Lacerations and hematomas
  - ○ Inversion of uterus
  - ○ Subinvolution of the uterus
  - ○ Retained placental fragments
  - ○ Coagulation disorders

- Subjective data
  - Increased vaginal bleeding
- Data collection findings
  - Soft, boggy uterus with possible displacement on palpation
  - Blood clots larger than a quarter
  - Perineal pad saturation in 15 min or less
  - Constant oozing, trickling, or frank flow of bright red blood from the vagina
  - Tachycardia, tachypnea, and hypotension
  - Skin that is pale, cool, and clammy with poor turgor and pale mucous membranes
  - Oliguria
- Laboratory tests
  - Hgb, Hct, and CBC with platelet count
  - Fibrinogen, fibrin split products, PT, and PTT
  - Blood type and antibody screen

Patient-Centered Care

- Nursing Care
  - Monitor vital signs.
  - Identify the source of bleeding.
    - Monitor fundus for height, firmness, and position. If the uterus is found to be boggy, massage it until it is firm in consistency.
    - Monitor bleeding for color and quantity.
    - Check for signs of bleeding from lacerations, episiotomy site, or hematomas.
  - Check bladder for distention.
  - Measure urinary output with an indwelling urinary catheter.
  - Monitor clients receiving IV fluid replacement with IV isotonic solutions, such as lactated Ringer's solution or 0.9% sodium chloride, crystalloid solutions, and blood or blood products (packed RBCs and fresh frozen plasma).
  - Provide oxygen to clients via nonrebreather mask to enhance oxygen delivery to the cells.
  - Monitor oxygen saturation with a pulse oximeter.
- Medications
  - Oxytocin (Pitocin)
    - Uterine stimulant to promote uterine contractions
  - Methylergonovine (Methergine)
    - Uterine stimulant to promote uterine contractions

○ Misoprostol (Cytotec)

  ▪ Uterine stimulant to promote uterine contractions

  ▪ Therapeutic intent – control postpartum hemorrhage

○ Carboprost (Hemabate, Dinoprostone)

  ▪ Uterine stimulant to promote uterine contractions

• Therapeutic Procedures

  ○ Surgical management can be necessary if bleeding persists.

• Care After Discharge

  ○ Client education

    ▪ Explain to clients to report excessive vaginal bleeding.

    ▪ Explain to clients to limit physical activity to conserve strength.

    ▪ Explain to clients to increase iron and protein intake to promote the rebuilding of RBC volume.

LACERATIONS AND HEMATOMAS

Overview

• Lacerations that occur during labor and birth consist of the tearing of soft tissues in the birth canal and adjacent structures including the cervical, vaginal, vulva, perineal, and/or rectal areas.

• An episiotomy can extend and become a third- or fourth-degree laceration.

• Hematomas can occur in the pelvic region or higher up in the vagina or broad ligament.

• Hematomas most often present with pain rather than visible bleeding.

Data Collection

• Risk Factors

  ○ Operative vaginal birth (forceps-assisted, vacuum-assisted birth)

  ○ Precipitous birth

  ○ Cephalopelvic disproportion

  ○ Size (macrosomic infant) and abnormal presentation or position of the fetus

  ○ Prolonged pressure of the fetal head on the vaginal mucosa

  ○ Previous scarring of the maternal birth canal from infection, injury, or operation

  ○ Vulvar, perineal, and vaginal varicosities

• Subjective Data

  ○ Persistent perineal or rectal pain or a feeling of pressure in the vagina

  ○ Difficulty voiding due to pressure on the urethra from a hematoma

- Data collection findings
  - Vaginal bleeding even though the uterus is firm and contracted
  - A continuous slow trickle of bright red blood from the vagina, laceration, or episiotomy
- Diagnostic procedures
  - Repair and suturing of the episiotomy or lacerations; ligation of the bleeding vessel or surgical incision for evacuation of the clotted blood from the hematoma

Patient-Centered Care

- Nursing Care
  - Monitor vital signs.
  - Inspect the cervix, vagina, perineum, and rectum for lacerations and/or hematomas.
  - Monitor bleeding.
  - Apply ice packs to treat small hematomas.
  - Administer pain medication.
  - Encourage sitz baths.
    - Encourage cleansing of the perineal area from front to back with a water bottle filled with warm tap water after voiding and defecation.

INFECTIONS (ENDOMETRITIS, MASTITIS, AND WOUND INFECTIONS)

Overview

- Postpartum infections are complications that can occur up to 28 days following childbirth, or a spontaneous or induced abortion. Fever of 38° C (100.4° F) or higher for 2 consecutive days during the first 10 days of the postpartum period is indicative of a postpartum infection and requires further investigation. The infection can be present in the bladder, uterus, wound, or breast of a postpartum client. The major complication of puerperal infection is septicemia.
- Uterine infection, mastitis, wound infection, and urinary tract infection are examples of postpartum infections. Early identification and prompt treatment are imperative to promote positive outcomes.

POSTPARTUM INFECTIONS	
Endometritis	› Infection of the uterine lining or endometrium.
	› Usually begins as a localized infection at the placental attachment site and can spread to include the entire uterine endometrium.
Mastitis	› Infection of the breast and is usually unilateral. An infected nipple fissure usually is the initial lesion, but the ductal system is involved next. Mastitis can progress to an abscess if untreated.
	› It occurs most commonly in mothers breastfeeding for the first time and well after the establishment of milk flow.
	› Staphylococcus aureus is usually the infecting organism.

POSTPARTUM INFECTIONS	
Wound Infections	› Sites of wound infections include cesarean incisions, episiotomies, lacerations, and/or any trauma wounds present in the birth canal following labor and birth. › Often develop after discharge to home.
Urinary tract infections (UTI)	› A potential complication of a UTI is the progression to pyelonephritis. › E. coli is often the infecting organism.

 View Image: Mastitis

Data Collection

- Risk Factors
  - Cesarean birth
  - Retained placental fragments and manual extraction of the placenta
  - Prolonged rupture of membranes, prolonged labor
  - Postpartum hemorrhage
  - Milk stasis from a blocked duct
  - Nipple trauma and cracked or fissured nipples
  - Decrease in breastfeeding frequency due to supplementation with bottle feeding
  - Poor hygiene with inadequate hand hygiene between handling perineal pads and breasts
  - Urinary bladder catheterization
    - Episiotomy, laceration, hematoma
- Subjective Data
  - Puerperal infections
    - Uterine tenderness, foul smelling, profuse lochia
    - Anorexia and nausea
    - Chills, fever, lethargy
  - Endometritis
    - Pelvic pain
  - Mastitis
    - Painful or tender, localized hard mass, and reddened area usually on one breast
  - Wound infection
    - Painful incision
  - Perineal discomfort
    - UTI
    - Reports of urgency, frequency, dysuria, and discomfort in the pelvic area

- Objective Data
  - Data collection findings
    - Puerperal infections
      - Elevated temperature of at least 38° C (100° F)
      - Tachycardia
    - Endometritis
      - Uterine tenderness and enlargement
      - Foul-smelling, profuse lochia
    - Mastitis
      - Axillary adenopathy in the affected side (enlarged tender axillary lymph nodes) with an area of inflammation that can be red, swollen, warm, and tender
    - Wound infection
      - Wound warmth, erythema, tenderness, pain, edema, seropurulent drainage, and wound dehiscence (separation of wound or incision edges).
    - UTI
      - Urine (hematuria, pyuria)
      - Costovertebral angle tenderness
  - Laboratory tests
    - Blood, intracervical, or intrauterine bacterial cultures to reveal the offending organism
    - WBC count (leukocytosis)
    - RBC sedimentation rate (distinctly increased)
    - RBC count (anemia)
    - Urinalysis positive for bacteria, blood

Patient-Centered Care

- Nursing Care
  - Obtain frequent vital signs and temperature.
  - Check fundal height, position, and consistency.
  - Determine the client's pain level.
  - Observe lochia for color, quantity, and consistency.
  - Inspect breasts, incisions, episiotomy, and lacerations.
    - Collect vaginal and blood cultures.
    - Monitor administration of IV fluids and antibiotics.
    - Encourage fluid intake of 2 to 3 L/day from food and beverage sources.
    - Administering analgesics as prescribed.
    - Reinforce good hand hygiene techniques.

- Encourage clients to maintain interaction with infants to facilitate bonding.

- Provide comfort measures such as warm blankets or warm or cool compresses, sitz baths, and perineal care.

- Perform wound care.

- Medications for endometritis

  - Clindamycin, cephalosporins, penicillins, and gentamicin

    - Broad-spectrum antibiotic therapy used in the treatment of bacterial infections.

  - Client education

    - Remind clients to take all the medication as prescribed.

    - Reinforce teaching with clients to notify the provider of the development of watery, bloody diarrhea.

- Care After Discharge

  - Client education

    - Encourage clients to practice thorough hand hygiene and good maternal perineal hygiene (changing perineal pads from front to back).

    - Encourage clients to consume a diet high in protein to promote tissue-healing.

    - Reinforce teaching with clients with mastitis to:

      - Use ice packs or warm packs on her affected breasts for discomfort.

      - Begin breastfeeding from the unaffected breast first to initiate the letdown reflex in the affected breast that is distended or tender.

      - Continue breastfeeding frequently (at least every 2 to 4 hr), especially on the affected side. Instruct clients to manually express breast milk or use a breast pump if breastfeeding is too painful. If an abscess forms, it can cause contamination of breast milk. If this occurs, breastfeeding should be stopped and the breasts pumped until resolved.

    - Reinforce teaching with clients who are breastfeeding to:

      - Perform hand hygiene prior to breastfeeding.

      - Change breast pads frequently.

      - Completely empty each breast during each feeding for prevention of milk stasis, which provides a medium for bacterial growth.

      - Allow nipples to air dry.

      - Wear a well-fitting bra for support.

      - Reinforce proper infant positioning and latching-on techniques, including both the nipple and the areola. The mother should release the infant's grasp on the nipple prior to removing the infant from the breast.

      - Encourage clients to get adequate rest and maintain a fluid intake of 2 to 3 L per day.

      - Instruct clients to report breast tenderness, redness, fever, malaise, urgency, frequency, dysuria, or perineal discomfort not relieved with analgesics.

      - Instruct clients to complete the entire course of antibiotics.

POSTPARTUM ADJUSTMENT AND MALADJUSTMENT

Overview

- Postpartum blues can occur in approximately 50% to 70% of women during the first few days after birth and generally continues for up to 10 days. Postpartum blues typically resolves in 10 days without intervention.

- Postpartum depression occurs within 4 weeks of delivery and is characterized by persistent feelings of sadness and intense mood swings. It occurs in 10% to 15% of new mothers and usually does not resolve without intervention. It is similar to nonpostpartum mood disorders.

- Postpartum psychosis develops within the first 2 weeks of the postpartum period. Clients who have a history of bipolar disorder are at a higher risk. The symptoms are severe and can include confusion, disorientation, auditory or visual hallucinations, delusions, obsessive behaviors, and paranoia. The client may attempt to harm herself or her infant.

  ○ The nurse should monitor clients for suicidal or delusional thoughts. The infant should be monitored for an inability of the mother to provide care for her newborn.

Data Collection

- Risk Factors
  ○ Hormonal changes with a rapid decline in estrogen and progesterone levels
  ○ "Difficult" infant temperament
  ○ Low socioeconomic status
  ○ Decreased social support system
  ○ Anxiety about assuming new role as a mother
  ○ Unplanned or unwanted pregnancy
  ○ History of previous depressive episode
  ○ Low self-esteem
  ○ Marital relationship problems

- Subjective Data
  ○ Postpartum blues
    ▪ Feelings of sadness
    ▪ Let-down feeling
    ▪ Fatigue, insomnia
    ▪ Restlessness
    ▪ Intense mood swings, emotional lability
    ▪ Anxiety and anger

- ○ Postpartum depression
  - ▪ Intense fears
  - ▪ Anger
  - ▪ Anxiety
  - ▪ Sadness that persists past the baby's first few weeks of life
  - ▪ Odd food cravings and binge eating with abnormal appetite
  - ▪ Pervasive sadness
  - ▪ Severe and labile mood swings
  - ▪ Sleep pattern disturbances
- ○ Postpartum psychosis
  - ▪ Deficits in judgment
  - ▪ Disorientation
  - ▪ Confusion
  - ▪ High levels of impulsivity
- • Objective Data
  - ○ Data collection findings
    - ▪ Postpartum blues
      - □ Crying
    - ▪ Postpartum depression
      - □ Pervasive sadness with severe and labile mood swings
      - □ Weight gain
      - □ Disinterest in the baby
    - ▪ Postpartum psychosis
      - □ Behaviors indicating hallucinations or delusional thoughts of self-harm or harming the infant

Patient-Centered Care

- • Nursing Care
  - ○ Monitor interactions between the mother and her newborn. Encourage bonding activities.
  - ○ Monitor client's mood and affect.
  - ○ Reinforce with clients that feeling down in the postpartum period is expected and self-limiting. Encourage clients to notify the provider if the condition persists.
  - ○ Encourage clients to communicate feelings, validate and address personal conflicts, and reinforce personal power and autonomy.
  - ○ Reinforce with clients the importance of adherence with any prescribed antidepressant medication regimen.

- Medications
  - Antidepressants may be prescribed by the provider if indicated based on the client's condition.
- Care After Discharge
  - Nursing actions
    - Schedule a follow-up visit prior to the traditional 6-week postpartum visit for clients who are at risk for developing postpartum depression.
    - Request a referral for a mental health consult if indicated.
    - Provide information about community resources such as La Leche League or support groups for new mothers.
  - Client education
    - Advise clients to get plenty of rest and to nap when the newborn sleeps.
    - Reinforce the importance of the client taking time out for herself.
    - Encourage clients to ask for help from family members.

APPLICATION EXERCISES

1. A nurse is caring for a postpartum client. Which of the following findings are the earliest indications of hypovolemia caused by hemorrhage?

    A. Increasing pulse and decreasing blood pressure

    B. Dizziness and increasing respiratory rate

    C. Cool, clammy skin and pale mucous membranes

    D. Altered mental status and level of consciousness

2. A nurse is providing care for a postpartum client who is experiencing a postpartum hemorrhage. Which of the following medications may be prescribed by the provider? (Select all that apply.)

    _____ A. Methylergonovine (Methergine)

    _____ B. Misoprostol (Cytotec)

    _____ C. Carboprost (Hemabate)

    _____ D. Hydralazine

    _____ E. Oxytocin (Pitocin)

3. A nurse is caring for a client who has disseminated intravascular coagulation (DIC). Which of the following postpartum complications is a risk factor for this client?

    A. Hemorrhage

    B. Thrombophlebitis

    C. Diabetes mellitus

    D. Hyperemesis gravidarum

4. A client who is breastfeeding has mastitis. Which of the following should the nurse reinforce to the client?

    A. Use a breast pump until the condition subsides, and stop breastfeeding.

    B. Nurse the infant only on the unaffected breast until resolved.

    C. Completely empty each breast at each feeding.

    D. Wear a breast binder until lactation has ceased.

5. A nurse is caring for a client who has urinary tract infection. Which of the following is the typical causative agent of infection?

    A. *Staphylococcus aureus*

    B. *E. coli*

    C. *Klebsiella pneumonia*

    D. *Clostridium perfringens*

6. A nurse educator is reviewing care of a client who has endometritis with a group of newly hired nurses. What should be included in the review? Use the ATI Active Learning Template: Systems Disorder to complete this item to include the following:

    A. Description of the Disorder

    B. Objective and Subjective Data: Describe at least three of each.

    C. Nursing Care: Describe at least three nursing interventions.

APPLICATION EXERCISES KEY

1. A. **CORRECT:** A rising pulse rate and decreasing blood pressure are often the first indications of inadequate blood volume.

    B. INCORRECT: Dizziness and increased respiratory rate are findings that occur in hypovolemia, but they are not the earliest indicators.

    C. INCORRECT: Skin that is cool, clammy, and pale along with pale mucous membranes are changes that occur in the physical status of a client who has decreased blood volume, but they are not the first indicators of inadequate blood volume.

    D. INCORRECT: Altered mental status and changes in level of consciousness are late manifestations of decreased blood volume, which leads to hypoxia and low oxygen saturation.

    (N) NCLEX® Connection: Physiological Adaptations, Alterations in Body Systems

2. A. **CORRECT:** Methylergonovine contracts the uterus and can be prescribed for the management of postpartum hemorrhage.

    B. **CORRECT:** Misoprostol contracts the uterus and can be prescribed for the management of postpartum hemorrhage.

    C. **CORRECT:** Carboprost contracts the uterus and can be prescribed for the management of postpartum hemorrhage.

    D. INCORRECT: Hydralazine is a vasodilator and is used in the management of pregnancy-induced hypertension.

    E. **CORRECT:** Oxytocin contracts the uterus and can be prescribed for the management of postpartum hemorrhage.

    (N) NCLEX® Connection: Pharmacological Therapies, Expected Actions/Outcomes

3. A. **CORRECT:** DIC can occur secondary in a client who has a postpartum hemorrhage.

    B. INCORRECT: Thrombophlebitis is not a risk factor for the development of DIC.

    C. INCORRECT: Diabetes mellitus is not a risk factor for the development of DIC.

    D. INCORRECT: Hyperemesis gravidarum is not a risk factor for the development of DIC.

    (N) NCLEX® Connection: Physiological Adaptations, Alterations in Body Systems

4.   A. INCORRECT: The nurse should instruct the client to continue breastfeeding.

     B. INCORRECT: The nurse should instruct the client to breastfeed, especially on the affected side.

     C. **CORRECT:** The nurse should instruct the client to completely empty each breast at each feeding for the prevention of milk stasis, which provides a medium for bacterial growth.

     D. INCORRECT: The nurse should instruct the client to wear a well-fitting bra, not one that is too tight or a binder.

     (N) NCLEX® Connection: Physiological Adaptations, Alterations in Body Systems

5.   A. INCORRECT: *Staphylococcus aureus* is usually the infecting organism in mastitis.

     B. **CORRECT:** *E. coli* is the usual causative agent associated with urinary tract infections.

     C. INCORRECT: *Klebsiella pneumonia* is not associated with urinary tract infections.

     D. INCORRECT: *Clostridium perfringens* is not associated with urinary tract infections.

     (N) NCLEX® Connection: Physiological Adaptations, Alterations in Body Systems

6.   *Using the ATI Active Learning Template: Systems Disorder*

     A. Description of the Disorder
        • Endometritis is an infection of the uterine lining or endometrium. It usually begins on the second to fifth postpartum day as a localized infection at the placental attachment site and spreads to include the entire endometrium. It is the most frequently occurring puerperal infection.

     B. Objective Data and Subjective Data
        • Objective Data
           ○ Uterine tenderness and enlargement
           ○ Dark, profuse lochia
           ○ Malodorous or purulent lochia
           ○ Temperature greater than 38° C (100.4° F) on the third or fourth postpartum day
           ○ Tachycardia
        • Subjective Data
           ○ Pelvic pain
           ○ Chills
           ○ Fatigue, loss of appetite

     C. Nursing Care
        • Collect vaginal and blood cultures.
        • Administer IV antibiotics as prescribed.
        • Administer analgesics as prescribed.
        • Reinforce teaching with client regarding hand hygiene techniques.
        • Encourage client interaction with her infant to facilitate bonding.

     (N) NCLEX® Connection: Physiological Adaptations, Alterations in Body Systems

UNIT 4   Newborn Nursing Care

CHAPTERS

› Newborn Data Collection
› Nursing Care of the Newborn
› Complications of the Newborn
› Baby-Friendly Care

NCLEX® CONNECTIONS

When reviewing the chapters in this unit, keep in mind the relevant sections of the NCLEX® outline, in particular:

Client Needs: Health Promotion and Maintenance

› Relevant topics/tasks include:

  » Aging Process

    › Provide care that meets the needs of the newborn less than 1 month old through the infant or toddler client through 2 years.

  » Ante/Intra/Postpartum and Newborn Care

    › Perform care of postpartum client.

    › Contribute to newborn plan of care.

    › Reinforce client teaching on infant care skills.

  » Data Collection Techniques

    › Collect data for health history.

    › Collect baseline physical data.

  » Developmental Stages and Transitions

    › Identify and report client deviations from expected growth and development.

    › Assist client with expected life transition.

Client Needs: Physiological Adaptation

› Relevant topics/tasks include:

  » Alterations in Body Systems

    › Identify signs and symptoms of an infection.

    › Provide care for a client experiencing complications of pregnancy/labor and/or delivery.

  » Fluid and Electrolyte Imbalances

    › Identify signs and symptoms of client fluid and/or electrolyte imbalances.

Client Needs: Pharmacological Therapies

› Relevant topics/tasks include:

  » Expected Actions/Outcomes

    › Apply knowledge of pathophysiology when addressing client pharmacological agents.

Client Needs: Reduction of Risk Potential

› Relevant topics/tasks include:

  » Potential for Complications of Diagnostic Tests/Treatments/Procedures

    › Implement measures to prevent complication of client condition or procedure.

UNIT 4   NEWBORN NURSING CARE

CHAPTER 14   Newborn Data Collection

Overview

- Apgar scoring, head-to-toe data collection (including vital signs and measurements), gestational age assessment, periods of adjustment to extrauterine life, and diagnostic and therapeutic procedures are components of newborn data collection.

- Newborn data collection occurs at birth (Apgar scoring, quick head-to-toe examination), upon admission into the nursery, and then before discharge.

- Equipment for Data Collection Following Birth

  ○ Bulb syringe – Used for suctioning excess mucus from the newborn's mouth and nose

  ○ Stethoscope with a pediatric head – Used to evaluate the newborn's heart rate, breath sounds, and bowel sounds

  ○ Axillary thermometer – Used to monitor the newborn's temperature

  ○ Blood pressure cuff (width-to-arm or -calf ratio approximately ½ to ¾) – For evaluation of the newborn's blood pressure

  ○ Scale with paper in place – Weight should include pounds, ounces, and grams

  ○ Tape measure with centimeters

  ○ Clean gloves – Used for examining newborns until the first bath is given

- Initial Data Collection

  ○ An Apgar score is assigned at 1 min and 5 min of life based on five assessment parameters.

SCORE	0	1	2
Heart rate	› Absent	› Less than 100	› Greater than 100
Respiratory rate	› Absent	› Slow, weak cry	› Good cry
Muscle tone	› Flaccid	› Some flexion	› Well-flexed
Reflex irritability	› None	› Grimace	› Cry
Color	› Blue, pale	› Pink body, cyanotic hands and feet (acrocyanosis)	› Completely pink

  ▪ 0 to 3 indicates severe distress
  ▪ 4 to 6 indicates moderate distress
  ▪ 7 to 10 indicates no distress

 View Video: Apgar Scoring

○ Head-to-toe exam of newborns within 24 hr of birth.

○ Obtain vital signs in the following sequence: respirations, heart rate, blood pressure, and temperature.

  ▪ Respiratory rate ranges from 30 to 60/min with short periods of apnea (less than 20 seconds). Abnormal findings include periods of apnea lasting longer than 20 seconds, crackles and wheezing (fluid or infection in the lungs), grunting, retractions, and nasal flaring (respiratory distress).

  ▪ Heart rate should be 100 to 160/min with brief fluctuations above and below this range depending on activity level (crying, sleeping). Apical pulse rate should be obtained for a full minute, preferably when newborns are sleeping. Place the stethoscope head on the fourth or fifth intercostal space at the left midclavicular line over the apex of the newborn's heart. Report heart murmurs.

  ▪ Blood pressure should be 60 to 80 mm Hg systolic and 40 to 50 mm Hg diastolic.

  ▪ Temperature should be 36.5° to 37.2° C (97.7 to 98.9° F) axillary. Take an initial rectal temperature per facility policy to check for anal abnormalities. Avoid routine rectal temperatures to prevent injury to rectal mucosa.

○ Obtain measurements by measuring the newborn's length from crown to heel of foot for length, and head circumference at greatest diameter (occipital to frontal). Measure the newborn's chest circumference beginning at the nipple line.

○ Physical exam from head to toe

  ▪ Posture

    ▫ Newborns should be lying in a curled-up position with arms and legs in moderate flexion.

  ▪ Skin

    ▫ Color should be pink or acrocyanotic with no jaundice present on the first day.

    ▫ Physiological jaundice appears by the third day, but should resolve within a few days.

    ▫ Good turgor is indicated by skin returning to its original state immediately when pinched.

    ▫ Texture should be dry, soft, and smooth showing good hydration. Cracks in hands and feet can be present. In full-term newborns, desquamation (peeling) occurs a few days after birth.

    ▫ Vernix caseosa (protective, thick, cheesy covering) amounts vary, with more present in the newborn's face, shoulders and back.

    ▫ Lanugo (fine downy hair) can be present and usually is found on the newborn's face, shoulders, and back.

    ▫ Normal deviations

      ▸ Milia (small raised white spots on the nose, chin, and forehead) can be present. These spots disappear spontaneously without treatment. (Caregivers should not squeeze the spots.)

      ▸ Mongolian spots (bluish purple spots of pigmentation) commonly are noted on the newborn's shoulders, back, and buttocks. These spots frequently are present on newborns who have dark skin. Be sure the parents are aware of Mongolian spots, and notify providers of the location and presence of them.

      ▸ Telangiectatic nevi (stork bites) are flat pink or red marks that easily blanch and are found on the newborn's back of the neck, nose, upper eyelids, and lower occipital area. They usually fade by the second year of life.

▸ Nevus flammeus (port wine stain) is a capillary angioma below the surface of the skin that is purple or red, varies in size and shape, is commonly seen on the face, and does not blanch or disappear.

▸ Erythema toxicum (erythema neonatorum) is a pink rash that appears suddenly anywhere on the body of a term newborn during the first 3 weeks. This is frequently referred to as newborn rash. No treatment is required.

View Images
› Mongolian Spots   › Telangiectatic Nevi

- Head
  □ Head circumference should be 2 to 3 cm larger than the chest circumference. A head circumference greater than or equal to 4 cm larger than the chest circumference can be an indication of hydrocephalus (excessive cerebral fluid within the brain cavity surrounding the brain). A head circumference less than or equal to 32 cm can be an indication of microcephaly (abnormally small head).

  □ The anterior fontanel should be approximately 5 cm and diamond shaped. The posterior fontanel is smaller and triangle shaped. Both fontanels should be soft and flat. The fontanels can bulge when the newborn cries, coughs, or vomits, and flat when the newborn is quiet. Bulging fontanels can indicate increased intracranial pressure, infection, or hemorrhage. Depressed fontanels can indicate dehydration.

  □ The sutures of newborns should be palpable, separated, and may be overlapping (molding), a normal occurrence resulting from head compression during labor.

  □ Caput succedaneum (localized swelling of the soft tissues of the scalp caused by pressure on the head during labor) is an expected finding that may be palpated as a soft edematous mass and can cross over the suture line. Caput succedaneum usually resolves in 3 to 4 days and does not require treatment.

  □ Cephalohematoma is a collection of blood between the periosteum and the skull bone that it covers. It does not cross the suture line. It results from trauma during birth, such as pressure of the fetal head against the maternal pelvis in a prolonged difficult labor or forceps delivery. It appears several hours or a day after birth and spontaneously resolves in 3 to 6 weeks.

View Images
› Caput Succedaneum   › Cephalohematoma

- Eyes
  □ Eyes should be symmetrical in size and shape.

  □ Each of the newborn's eyes and the space between them should equal one-third of the total distance between the outer canthus of both eyes. Epicanthal folds, when present with other findings, can indicate chromosomal disorders such as Down syndrome.

  □ Occasional tears can be present.

  □ Subconjunctival hemorrhages can be present.

  □ Pupillary and red reflex should be present.

  □ Eyeball movement will demonstrate random, jerky movements.

- Ears
  - When examining the placement of the newborn's ears, draw an imaginary line through the inner to the outer canthus of the newborn's eye. The eye should be even with the upper tip of the pinna of the newborn's ear. Ears that are low-set can indicate a chromosomal disorder, mental retardation, or kidney disorder.
  - Cartilage should be firm and well-formed. Lack of cartilage indicates prematurity.
  - Newborns should respond to voices and other sounds.
  - Inspect the newborn's ears for skin tags.
- Nose
  - Nose should be midline; can also be flat and broad with lack of a bridge.
  - Some mucus, but with no drainage.
  - Newborn should sneeze to clear his nose.
- Mouth
  - The lip movements should be symmetrical with strong suck reflex.
  - Saliva should be scant. Excessive saliva can indicate a tracheoesophageal fistula.
  - Epstein pearls (small white cysts found on the gums and at the junction of the soft and hard palates) are normal in newborns. They result from the accumulation of epithelial cells and disappear a few weeks after birth.
  - The tongue should move freely, be symmetrical in shape, and not protrude. A protruding tongue can indicate a chromosomal disorder.
  - The soft and hard palate should be intact.
  - The gums and tongue should be pink. White plaques on cheeks or tongue that bleed if touched can indicate thrush, a fungal infection caused by *Candida albicans*, sometimes acquired from the mother's vaginal secretions.
- Neck
  - The neck should be short and thick, surrounded by skin folds, and exhibit no webbing.
  - The neck should move freely from side to side and up and down.
  - Absence of head control can indicate prematurity or chromosomal disorder.
- Chest
  - The chest should be almost circular, barrel-shaped.
  - Respirations are primarily diaphragmatic without retractions.
  - Clavicles should be intact.
  - The nipples should be prominent, well-formed, and symmetrical with breast nodules approximately 6 mm. Can be edematous related to maternal hormones.
- Abdomen
  - The umbilical cord should have two arteries and one vein.
  - The umbilical cord should be odorless and exhibit no intestinal structures.
  - The abdomen should be round, dome-shaped, and nondistended.
  - Bowel sounds should be present within minutes following birth.

- Anogenital
  - The anus should be present, patent, and not covered by a membrane.
  - The genitalia of a male newborn should include rugae on the scrotum, testes descended into the scrotum, and the urinary meatus located at penile tip.
  - The genitalia of a female newborn should include labia majora covering the labia minora and clitoris. Female genitalia are usually edematous, with a hymenal tag present and possible vaginal blood-tinged discharge, caused by maternal pregnancy hormones.
  - Urine should be passed within 24 hr after birth. Uric acid crystals will produce a rust color in the urine the first couple of days of life.
  - Meconium should be passed within 24 to 48 hr after birth.
- Extremities
  - Full range and symmetry of motion, spontaneous movements, and equal length.
  - Extremities should be flexed with resistance to extension of his extremities.
  - No click should be heard when abducting the hips of a newborn.
  - Symmetrical gluteal folds, bowed legs, and flat feet.
  - Two-thirds of the soles of the feet should be well-lined.
  - The nail beds should be pink, and no extra digits present.
- Spine
  - The newborn's spine should be straight, flat, midline, and easily flexed.
  - Reflexes

REFLEX	EXPECTED FINDING	EXPECTED AGE
Sucking and rooting reflex	› This reflex is elicited by stroking the newborn's cheek or edge of his mouth. The newborn will turn his head toward the side that is touched and start to suck.	› Birth to 4 months; may persist up to 1 year
Palmar grasp	› This reflex is elicited by placing an object in the newborn's palm. The newborn will grasp the object.	› Birth to 3 months
Plantar grasp	› This reflex is elicited by touching the sole of the newborn's foot. The newborn will respond by curling his toes downward.	› Birth to 8 months
Moro reflex	› This reflex is elicited by allowing the head and trunk of the newborn in a semisitting position to fall backward to an angle of at least 30°. The newborn's arms and legs will extend symmetrically and then abduct while his fingers spread to form a "C."	› Birth to 4 months
Startle reflex	› This reflex is elicited by clapping hands or by a loud noise. The newborn will abduct arms at the elbows, and the hands will remain clenched.	› Birth to 4 months

REFLEX	EXPECTED FINDING	EXPECTED AGE
Tonic neck reflex (fencer position)	› This reflex is elicited by turning a newborn's head to one side. The newborn will respond by extending his arm and leg on that side, and flex his arm and leg on the opposite side.	› Birth to 3 to 4 months
Babinski's reflex	› This reflex is elicited by stroking the outer edge of the sole of a newborn's foot, moving up toward his toes. The newborn's toes will fan upward and out.	› Birth to 1 year
Stepping	› This reflex is elicited by holding the newborn upright with his feet touching a flat surface. The newborn will respond with stepping movements.	› Birth to 4 weeks

View Image: Babinski's Reflex

- Senses
  - Vision – The newborn should be able to focus on objects 8 to 12 inches away from his face. This is approximately the distance from the mother's face when the newborn is breastfeeding. The newborn's eyes are sensitive to light, so newborns prefer dim lighting. Pupils are reactive to light, and the blink reflex is easily stimulated. The newborn can track high-contrast objects, and prefers black and white and patterns.
  - Hearing – Similar to that of an adult once the amniotic fluid drains from the ears.
  - Touch – Newborns should respond to tactile messages of pain and touch.
  - Taste – Newborns can taste and prefer sweets over salty, sour, or bitter.
  - Smell – Newborns have a highly developed sense of smell, prefer sweet smells, and can recognize the scent of their mother.
- Gestational Age Assessment
  - Gestational age assessment is performed within the first 48 hr of life. For infants with a gestational age of 26 weeks or less, it should be performed at a postnatal age of less than 12 hr. This examination involves taking measurements of newborns and the use of the New Ballard Scale. This scale provides an estimation of gestational age and a baseline to determine growth and development.
  - The expected ranges of physical measurements
    - Weight – 2,500 to 4,000 g (Weigh newborns at the same time daily.)
    - Length – 45 to 55 cm (18 to 22 in)
    - Head circumference – 32 to 36.8 cm (12.6 to 14.5 in)
    - Chest circumference – 30 to 33 cm (12 to 13 in)

- New Ballard Scale – A newborn maturity rating scale that evaluates neuromuscular and physical maturity. Each individual assessment parameter displays at least six ranges of development along a continuum. Each range of development within the examination is assigned a number value from -1 to 5. The totals are added to give a maturity rating in weeks gestation. (A score of 35 indicates 38 weeks of gestation.)
- Neuromuscular maturity determines:
  - Posture ranging from fully extended to fully flexed (0 to 4).
  - Square window formation with the neonate's wrist (-1 to 4).
  - Arm recoil, where the neonate's arm is passively extended and spontaneously returns to flexion (0 to 4).
  - Popliteal angle, which is the degree of the angle to which the newborn's knees can extend (-1 to 5).
  - Scarf sign, which is crossing the neonate's arm over the chest (-1 to 4).
  - Heel to ear, which is how far the neonate's heels reach to her ears (-1 to 4).
- Physical maturity determines:
  - Skin texture, ranging from sticky and transparent, to leathery, cracked, and wrinkled (-1 to 5).
  - Lanugo presence and amount, ranging from none, sparse, abundant, thinning, bald, or mostly bald (-1 to 4).
  - Plantar surface creases, ranging from less than 40 to 50 mm, to creases over the entire sole (-1 to 4).
  - Breast tissue amount, ranging from imperceptible to full areola with a 5 to 10 mm bud (-1 to 4).
  - Eyes and ears for amount of eye opening and ear cartilage present (-1 to 4).
  - Genitalia development, ranging from flat smooth scrotum to pendulous testes with deep rugae for males (-1 to 4), and prominent clitoris with flat labia to the labia majora covering the labia minora and clitoris for females (-1 to 4).
- Following the physical examination of newborns, classification of newborns by gestational age and birth weight is then determined.
  - Appropriate for gestational age (AGA) – Weight is between the 10th and 90th percentile.
  - Small for gestational age (SGA) – Weight is below the 10th percentile.
  - Large for gestational age (LGA) – Weight is above the 90th percentile.
  - Low birth weight (LBW) – A weight of 2,500 g or less at birth.
    - Term – Birth between the beginning of week 38 and prior to the end of 42 weeks of gestation
    - Preterm or premature – Born prior to the completion of 37 weeks of gestation
    - Postterm (postdate) – Born after the completion of 42 weeks of gestation
    - Postmature – Born after the completion of 42 weeks of gestation with signs of placental insufficiency

- Periods of Adjustment
  - ○ Observe for periods of reactivity in newborns during the first 6 to 8 hr of life.
    - ▪ First period of reactivity – Newborns are alert, may have spontaneous startles, tremors, crying, and head movements from side to side, and have a rapid heartbeat and respiratory rate. Heart rate can be as high as 160 to 180/min, but will stabilize at a baseline of 100 to 120/min. This period lasts up to 30 min after birth. This is the optimal time for bonding and breastfeeding to take place.
    - ▪ Period of relative inactivity – Newborns will become quiet and begin rest and sleep. The newborn's heart rate and respirations will decrease. This period begins after the first period of reactivity and lasts from 60 to 100 min.
    - ▪ Second period of reactivity – Brief periods of tachycardia and tachypnea occur, associated with increased muscle tone, changes in skin color, and mucus production. Meconium is commonly passed at this time. This period usually occurs 2 to 8 hr after birth and can last 10 min to several hours.
- Diagnostic and Therapeutic Procedures Following Birth
  - ○ Laboratory tests
    - ▪ Hgb, Hct, and WBC
    - ▪ Blood type, Rh-status
    - ▪ Glucose for hypoglycemia, per facility policy or order
    - ▪ Serum bilirubin per facility policy or prescription

    - ▪ Phenylketonuria (PKU) testing is required by all states. PKU is a defect in protein metabolism in which the accumulation of the amino acid phenylalanine can result in mental retardation (treatment in the first 2 months of life can prevent retardation). A capillary heel stick should be done 24 hr following birth. For results to be accurate, newborns must receive formula or breast milk for at least 24 hr. If newborns are discharged before 24 hr of age, the test should be repeated in 1 to 2 weeks.
    - ▪ Other genetic testing that can be done includes galactosemia, cystic fibrosis, maple syrup urine disease, hypothyroidism, and sickle cell disease.
    - ▪ Perform heel stick to obtain blood for testing.
      - □ Warm the newborn's heel first to increase circulation and eliminate or decrease the pain associated with a heel stick.
      - □ Cleanse the newborn's heel with alcohol or skin antiseptic, and allow for drying.
      - □ Use a spring-activated lancet so that the skin incision is made quickly and painlessly.
      - □ Use the outer aspect of the heel, and do not let the lancet go any deeper than 2.4 mm, to prevent necrotizing osteochondritis resulting from penetration of bone with the lancet.
      - □ Obtain the specimen.
      - □ Apply pressure with dry gauze (do not use alcohol as it will cause bleeding to continue) until bleeding stops and cover with an adhesive bandage.
      - □ Cuddle and comfort newborns when the procedure is completed to reassure newborns and promote feelings of safety.

EXPECTED LABORATORY VALUES			
Hgb	14.5 to 22.5 g/dL	Platelets	150,000 to 300,000/mm^3
Hct	48% to 69%	Glucose	40 to 60 mg/dL
RBC count	4,800,000 to 7,100,000/mm^3	Bilirubin	0 to 6 mg/dL on day 1
Leukocytes	9,000 to 30,000/mm^3		8 mg/dL or less on day 2
			12 mg/dL or less on days 2 to 5

- Diagnostic Procedures
  - Most states have enacted legislation mandating universal hearing screening. It is performed routinely in other states. Most newborns in the United States (95%) are screened for hearing loss before leaving the hospital.
  - Pulse oximetry screening at 24 to 48 hr per facility protocol.

APPLICATION EXERCISES

1. A nurse is caring for a newborn in the nursery. The newborn weighs 3,200 g and is in the 60th percentile for weight. Apgar scores are 9 and 10 at 1 and 5 min of age. Vital signs are temperature 37.2° C (99.1° F) axillary, heart rate 160/min, respirations 48/min, length 50.8 cm (20 in), head circumference 35 cm (14 in), and chest circumference 33 cm (13 in). Which of the following is an appropriate classification for the newborn based on weight and gestational age?

   A. Low birth weight (LBW)

   B. Appropriate for gestational age (AGA)

   C. Small for gestational age (SGA)

   D. Large for gestational age (LGA)

2. A nurse is collecting data from a newborn and observes small white bumps noted on the bridge of the nose. The nurse should document this finding as which of the following?

   A. Erythema toxicum

   B. Epstein's pearls

   C. Mongolian spots

   D. Milia spots

3. A nurse is assisting a registered nurse with the care of a newborn following a low forceps vaginal delivery. Five minutes after birth, the newborn's heart rate is 110/min. Which of the following Apgar heart rate scores should the newborn receive?

   A. 0

   B. 1

   C. 2

   D. 3

4. A nurse is checking the reflexes of a newborn. Which of the following should the nurse perform to elicit the startle reflex?

   A. Hold the newborn in a semisitting position, then allow the newborn's head and trunk to fall backward.

   B. Make a loud noise such as clapping hands together over the newborn's crib.

   C. Stimulate the pads of the newborn's hands with a stroking touch.

   D. Stimulate the soles of the newborn's feet on the outer lateral surface of each foot.

5. A nurse is assisting with the admission of a newborn to the nursery. Which of the following findings indicate that a newborn is experiencing difficulty adapting to extrauterine life? (Select all that apply.)

_____ A. Grunting

_____ B. Retractions

_____ C. Nasal flaring

_____ D. Apnea for 10-second periods

_____ E. Respiratory rate 55/min

6. A nurse in the nursery is admitting a newborn 2 hr following birth. What nursing actions should the nurse use to evaluate newborn physical development? Use the ATI Active Learning Template: Growth and Development to complete this item to include the following:

A. Physical Development:
  • Describe at least three tools for examination.
  • Describe four reflex responses present at birth and how they are elicited.
  • Describe newborn heart rate and how it is determined.

APPLICATION EXERCISES KEY

1. A. INCORRECT: A LBW newborn would weigh less than 2,500 grams.

    B. **CORRECT:** An AGA newborn's weight is between the 10th and 90th percentile, so this is the proper classification.

    C. INCORRECT: A SGA newborn's weight is below the 10th percentile

    D. INCORRECT: A LGA newborn's weight is above the 90th percentile.

    Ⓝ NCLEX® Connection: Health Promotion and Maintenance, Data Collection Techniques

2. A. INCORRECT: Erythema toxicum is a transient maculopapular rash seen in newborns.

    B. INCORRECT: Epstein's pearls are small white nodules that appear on the roof of a newborn's mouth.

    C. INCORRECT: Mongolian spots are dark bluish, purple areas noted on the shoulders, back, and buttocks of the newborn.

    D. **CORRECT:** Milia are small white bumps that occur on the nose due to clogged sebaceous glands.

    Ⓝ NCLEX® Connection: Health Promotion and Maintenance, Data Collection Techniques

3. A. INCORRECT: A 0 heart rate score is given for an absent heart rate at 5 min.

    B. INCORRECT: A 1 heart rate score is given for a heart rate less than 100/min at 5 min.

    C. **CORRECT:** The 5 min heart rate score should be two because the heart rate is greater than 100/min.

    D. INCORRECT: The Apgar score is 0, 1, or 2 for each individual sign of the newborn's physiologic state.

    Ⓝ NCLEX® Connection: Health Promotion and Maintenance, Data Collection Techniques

4. A. INCORRECT: Holding the newborn in a semisitting position and then allowing the head and trunk to fall backward elicits the moro reflex.

    B. **CORRECT:** Clapping of the hands will elicit the startle reflex in the newborn.

    C. INCORRECT: Stimulating the pads of the newborn's hands will elicit the grasp reflex.

    D. INCORRECT: Stimulating the outer lateral portion of the newborn's soles will elicit Babinski's reflex.

    Ⓝ NCLEX® Connection: Health Promotion and Maintenance, Data Collection Techniques

5.   A. **CORRECT:** Grunting is a sign of respiratory distress in the newborn.

B. **CORRECT:** Retractions are a sign of respiratory distress in the newborn.

C. **CORRECT:** Nasal flaring is a sign of respiratory distress in the newborn.

D. INCORRECT: Periods of apnea lasting less than 15 seconds are normal.

E. INCORRECT: Normal respiratory rate for a newborn increases from 30 to 60/min with short periods of apnea (less than 15 seconds).

Ⓝ NCLEX® Connection: Health Promotion and Maintenance, Developmental Stages and Transitions

6.   *Using the ATI Active Learning Template: Growth and Development*

A. Physical Development
- Assessment tools
  - Brief initial systems examination
  - Gestational age assessment
    - Physical measurements
    - New Ballard Scale
  - Vital signs
  - Head-to-toe physical examination
- Reflexes
  - Sucking and rooting – Turns head to side that is touched and begins to suck when cheek or edge of mouth is stroked.
  - Palmar grasp – Grasps object when placed in palm.
  - Plantar grasp – Toes curl downward when sole of the foot is touched.
  - Moro – Arms and legs symmetrically extend and then abduct while fingers spread to form a "C" when infant's head and trunk are allowed to fall backward to an angle of at least 30°.
  - Tonic neck (fencer position) – Extends arm and leg on same side when head is turned to that side, and flexes arm and leg of opposite side.
  - Babinski's – Toes fan upward and out when outer edge of sole of foot is stroked, moving up toward toes.
  - Stepping – Makes stepping movements when held upright with feet touching flat surface.
- Heart rate
  - 100 to 160/min with brief fluctuations above and below, depending on activity level.
  - When newborn is sleeping, place pediatric stethoscope head on fourth or fifth intercostal space at the left midclavicular line over apex of the heart. Listen for a full minute.
  - Note any murmurs.

Ⓝ NCLEX® Connection: Health Promotion and Maintenance, Data Collection Techniques

chapter 15

Overview

- Nurses play an important role in the care of newborns after birth. Initial nursing care includes maintaining a patent airway, monitoring vital signs, ensuring proper identification, maintaining thermoregulation, monitoring elimination patterns, preventing infection, and reinforcing discharge teaching for parents.

Low-Risk Newborn

- Initial Nursing Care

  - Maintain a patent airway. Keep the bulb syringe with newborns, and use it to keep nasal passages clear.

  - Check vital signs at admission/birth and every 30 min x 2, every 1 hr x 2, and then every 8 hr. (BP is not done unless cardiac problems are suspected.)

  - Monitor newborns for manifestations of respiratory complications.

    - Bradypnea – respirations less than 25/min

    - Tachypnea – respirations greater than 60/min

    - Abnormal breath sounds – expiratory grunting, crackles, and wheezes

    - Respiratory distress – nasal flaring, retractions, grunting, and labored breathing

  - Obtain daily weights.

    - Ensure proper identification.

  - Identification bands are applied to newborns, usually one on an ankle and one on a wrist, immediately after birth with corresponding bands for mother and significant other, if present. These bands can have permanent locks that must be cut to be removed. Identification bands should include the newborn's name, sex, date, time of birth, and mother's hospital number. In addition, the newborn's footprints and mother's thumbprints can be taken. The above information is included with the footprint sheet as well.

    - Each time the newborn is taken to his mother, the identification band should be verified against the mother's identification band.

    - All facility staff who assist in caring for newborns are required to wear picture identification badges.

    - Newborns are not to be given to anyone who does not have a picture identification badge that distinguishes that person as a staff member of the facility maternal-newborn unit.

    - Many facilities have locked maternal-newborn units that require staff to permit entrance or exit. Some facilities have a sensor device on the ID band or umbilical cord clamp that sounds an alarm if the newborn is removed from the facility.

- ○ Maintain thermoregulation
  - ▪ Monitor for manifestations of hypothermia.
    - □ Axillary temperature less than 36.5° C (97.7° F)
    - □ Cyanosis
    - □ Increased respiratory rate
  - ▪ Interventions to maintain thermoregulation
    - □ Maintain temperature between 36.5° C (97.7° F) and 37° C (98.6° F).
      - ▸ To prevent heat loss from conduction, preheat a radiant warmer and warm a stethoscope and other instruments before use, pad a scale with paper before weighing newborns, and place newborns directly on the mother's chest and cover with a warm blanket.
      - ▸ To prevent heat loss from convection, place the newborn's bassinet out of the direct line of a fan or air conditioning vent, swaddle newborns in a blanket, and keep the newborn's head covered. Perform procedures under a radiant heat source.
      - ▸ To prevent heat loss of evaporation, rub newborns dry with a warm sterile blanket immediately after delivery. Perform the initial bath when the newborn's skin temperature is 36.5° C (97.7° F). Perform under a radiant heat source. Expose only one body part at a time, washing and drying thoroughly.
      - ▸ To prevent heat loss from radiation, keep the newborn and examining tables away from windows and air conditioners.
  - ▪ Gloves should be worn until the newborn's first bath to avoid exposure to body secretions.
- ○ Provide nutrition immediately following birth.
  - ▪ Initiate breastfeeding as soon as possible after birth to promote maternal-newborn bonding.
  - ▪ Start formula feeding at about 2 to 4 hr of age. A few sips of sterile water can be given to check sucking and swallowing reflexes and ensure that there are no anomalies, such as a tracheoesophageal fistula, prior to starting formula feeding.
    - □ Feed newborns on demand, which is normally every 2 to 3 hr for breastfed newborns and 3 to 4 hr for bottle-fed newborns.
    - □ Monitor and document feedings per facility protocol.
    - □ Expect weight loss of 5% to 10% immediately after birth, which should be regained 10 to 14 days after birth.
  - ▪ Position newborns supine, "back to sleep," to decrease the risk of sudden infant death syndrome.
  - ▪ Monitor and document elimination patterns.
    - □ Newborns should void once within 24 hr of birth. They should void 6 to 10 times a day after 4 days of life.
  - ▪ Monitor and document the newborn's output.
    - □ Meconium should be passed within the first 24 hr after birth. The newborn will then continue to stool 3 to 4 times a day depending on whether he is being breast- or bottle-fed.
    - □ The stools of newborns who are breastfed can appear yellow and seedy. These stools are lighter in color and looser than the stools of newborns who are formula-fed.

- Keep the newborn's perineal area clean and dry.

  □ Wash the newborn's perineal area after each diaper change with clear water, or water and a mild soap. Avoid diaper wipes with alcohol. Pat dry, and apply triple antibiotic ointment, petroleum jelly, or zinc oxide, per facility protocol.

- Prevent infection by providing newborns their own bassinet equipped with a thermometer, diapers, T-shirts, and bathing supplies. Have all personnel caring for a newborn scrub with antimicrobial soap from elbows to fingertips before entering the nursery. Nurses should use proper hand hygiene when caring for newborns. Use cover gowns or special uniforms to avoid direct contact with clothes.

- Monitor the umbilical cord. Report a cord that is moist and red, has a foul odor, or has purulent drainage. Remove cord clamp before discharge.

- Provide family education and promotion of parent-newborn attachment.

  □ Provide family education while performing all nursing care. Encourage family involvement, allowing the mother and family to perform newborn care with direct supervision and support by the nurse.

  □ Encourage mothers and family to hold the newborn so that they can experience eye-to-eye contact and interaction.

- Laboratory tests

  - Blood glucose levels

  - Bilirubin level – direct and indirect if jaundice is present

  - Blood test for genetic screening – All states require testing for phenylketonuria (PKU) and hypothyroidism. Other genetic disorders that can be screened for include galactosemia, cystic fibrosis, and maple syrup urine disease. Blood samples are taken at least 24 hr after the first feeding.

- Diagnostic tests

  - Hearing screening – Newborns are screened for hearing loss with otoacoustic emissions testing and/or auditory brainstem response. Failure of these screening tests necessitates further testing to make a conclusive diagnosis.

- Medications

  - Erythromycin (Romycin)

    - Prophylactic eye care is the mandatory instillation of antibiotic ointment into the newborn's eyes to prevent ophthalmia neonatorum. Infections can be transmitted during descent through the birth canal. Ophthalmia neonatorum is caused by *Neisseria gonorrhoeae* or *Chlamydia trachomatis* and can cause blindness in the newborn.

    - Nursing considerations and client education

      □ Erythromycin is the medication of choice.

      □ Apply within 1 to 2 hr of birth.

      □ Use a single-dose unit to avoid cross-contamination between newborns.

      □ Apply a 1 to 2 cm ribbon of erythromycin ointment to the lower conjunctival sac of each eyes starting from the inner canthus and moving outward.

    - Client education

      □ A possible adverse reaction is chemical conjunctivitis, which can cause redness, swelling, drainage, and temporarily blurred vision for 24 to 48 hr. Reassure parents that this will resolve on its own.

Vitamin K (Aquamephyton)

- This vitamin injection is administered to prevent hemorrhagic disorders. Vitamin K is not produced in the gastrointestinal tract of the newborn until around day 8. Vitamin K is produced in the colon by bacteria that forms once formula or breast milk is introduced into the gut of the newborn.

  - Nursing considerations

    □ Administer 0.5 to 1 mg IM into the vastus lateralis (where muscle development is adequate) within 1 hr after birth.

○ Hepatitis B vaccination

  - This immunization provides protection for the newborn against hepatitis B.

  - Nursing considerations

    □ This immunization is recommended to be given to all newborns.

    □ For newborns born to healthy women, recommended dosage schedule is at birth, 1 month, and 6 months.

    □ For women infected with hepatitis B, hepatitis B immunoglobulin (HBIG) and with the hepatitis B vaccine are given within 12 hr of birth. The hepatitis B vaccine is given alone at 1, 2, and 12 months.

    □ Do not give vitamin K and the hepatitis B injections in the same thigh. Alternate sites.

○ Triple dye

  - Topical antimicrobial can be used for umbilical cord care.

  - Nursing considerations

    □ Care for the cord as prescribed. This can include applying triple dye to the umbilical stump or cleansing with sterile water, as recommended by the Association of Women's Health, Obstetrics and Neonatal Nurses. The cord should be kept clean and dry to prevent infection.

  - Therapeutic procedures

    □ Heel stick blood samples are obtained for blood glucose and bilirubin levels and genetic screening.

  - Nursing actions

    □ Warm the newborn's heel to increase circulation.

    □ Cleanse the newborn's heel with the appropriate antiseptic and allow to dry.

    □ Use a spring-activated lancet to puncture the skin at the outer aspect of the heel, no deeper than 2.4 mm.

    □ Follow facility protocol for specimen collection, equipment to be used, and labeling of specimens.

    □ Apply pressure with dry gauze (do not use alcohol, as it will cause bleeding to continue) until bleeding stops, and cover with an adhesive bandage.

    □ Cuddle and comfort the newborn when the procedure is completed to reassure the newborn and promote feelings of safety.

Q
PCC

- Care of the Newborn at Home
  - ○ Reinforce teaching to parents regarding home care of newborns. Determine previous newborn experience and knowledge, social support available, and educational needs.
  - ○ Crying
    - Inform parents that newborns cry when they are hungry, overstimulated, wet, cold, hot, tired, bored, or need to be burped. Assure the mother that in time, she will learn what her newborn's cry means. Instruct parents not to feed newborns every time they cry. Overfeeding can lead to stomach aches and diarrhea. It is okay to let a newborn cry for short periods of time.
  - ○ Quieting techniques
    - Swaddling
    - Close skin contact
    - Nonnutritive sucking
    - Rhythmic noises to simulate womb sounds
    - Movement (car ride, vibrating chair, infant swing, rocking newborn)
    - Placing the newborn on his stomach across a holder's lap while bouncing legs
    - En face
    - Stimulation
  - ○ Sleep-wake cycle
    - Instruct parents that most newborns sleep 16 out of every 24 hr the first week at home and sleep 2 to 3 hr at a time. Remind parents to place newborns in the supine position for sleeping.
    - Tell parents to keep the newborn's environment quiet and dark at night.
    - Discourage parents from allowing newborns in their bed.
    - Encourage parents to establish a predictable routine, such as bringing newborns out into the center of the action in the afternoon and keeping them there for the rest of the evening. Bathe newborns right before bedtime to provide comfort, give the last feeding around 11 p.m., and then place into a crib or bassinet.
    - Suggest that parents keep a small nightlight on to avoid having to turn on bright lights when giving nighttime feedings and changing diapers. Encourage parents to speak softly and handle newborns gently so that they go back to sleep easily.
  - ○ Oral and nasal suctioning
    - Reinforce to the parents to use a bulb syringe to suction any excess mucus from the newborn's nose and mouth.
    - Suction the newborn's mouth first and then the nose, one nostril at a time.
    - Compress the bulb syringe before inserting it into the newborn's mouth or nose.
    - When suctioning the newborn's mouth, always insert the bulb syringe on the sides of his mouth, not in the middle. To avoid eliciting the newborn's gag reflex, do not touch the back of the throat.

○ Positioning and holding the newborn

■ Reinforce to the parents that newborns have minimal head control. The head must be supported whenever newborns are lifted, especially because the head is larger than the rest of the body.

■ Instruct the parents in four basic ways to hold newborns.

▫ Cradle hold – Cradle the newborn's head in the bend of the elbow. This permits eye-to-eye contact (good for feeding).

▫ Upright position – Hold newborns upright and faced toward the holder while supporting the head, upper back, and buttocks (good for burping).

▫ Football hold – Support half of the newborn's body in the holder's forearm, with the newborn's head and neck resting in the palm of the hand (good for shampooing and breastfeeding).

▫ Colic hold – Place newborns face-down along the holder's forearm with the hand firmly between the newborn's legs. The newborn's cheek should be by the holder's elbow on the outside. Newborns should be able to see the ground, and the holder's arm should be close to their body, using it to brace and steady newborns (good for quieting a newborn who is fussy).

○ Bathing

■ Instruct the parents to:

▫ Cleanse the newborn's face, perineal area, and skin folds daily. Completely bathe the newborn 2 to 3 times per week using mild soap without hexachlorophene.

▫ Wash the area around the cord, taking care not to get it wet.

▫ Cleanse from the cleanest to dirtiest part of the newborn's body, beginning with his eyes, face, and head. Then proceed to the chest, arms, and legs. Wash the groin area last.

▫ Do not immerse newborns until the umbilical cord has fallen off, and until the circumcision has healed on males.

▫ Bathe newborns before a feeding to prevent spitting up or vomiting.

▫ Organize all equipment so that newborns are not left unattended in the water. Never leave newborns alone in the tub or sink.

▫ Make sure the hot water heater is set at 49° C (120.2° F) or less and that the room is warm. Bath water should be 36.6° to 37.2° C (97.8° to 99° F). Test the water for comfort on inner wrist prior to bathing newborns.

▫ Avoid drafts or chilling of newborns. Expose only the body part being bathed, and dry newborns thoroughly.

▫ Clean the newborn's eyes using a clean portion of the washcloth, and use clear water to clean each eye. Move from the inner to the outer canthus.

▫ Wrap the newborn in a towel and swaddle him in a football hold to shampoo his head.

▫ Rinse shampoo from the newborn's head, and dry to avoid chilling.

▫ To cleanse an uncircumcised penis of male newborns, wash with soap and water and rinse the penis. The foreskin should not be forced back, or constriction can result.

▫ In female newborns, wash the vulva by wiping from front to back to prevent contamination of the vagina or urethra from rectal bacteria.

▫ Do not use lotions, oils, or powders, because they can alter a newborn's skin, provide a medium for bacterial growth, or cause an allergic reaction. Powders also can be inhaled, leading to respiratory issues.

○ Feeding

- Nutritional requirements

  □ Fluid intake of 100 to 140 mL/kg/24 hr. Newborns should not be given water supplements because they receive enough water from breast milk or formula.

  □ For the first 3 months, newborns require 110 kcal/kg/day. From 3 to 6 months, the requirement decreases to 100 kcal/kg/day. Both breast milk and formula provide 20 kcal/oz. Expect newborns to gain 110 to 200 g/week for the first 3 months.

  □ Carbohydrates should make up 40% to 50% of the newborn's total caloric intake.

  □ At least 15% of calories must come from fat (triglycerides). The fat in breast milk is easier to digest than the fat in cow's milk.

  □ For adequate growth and development, newborns must receive 2.25 to 4 g/kg of protein per day. (For infants younger than 6 months, the average daily recommended intake for protein is 9.1 g/day).

  □ The mineral content of commercial newborn formula and breast milk is adequate, except for iron and fluoride.

    ▸ Iron is low in all forms of milk, but it is absorbed better from breast milk. Newborns who only breastfeed for the first 6 months maintain adequate Hgb levels and do not need any additional iron supplementation. After 6 months of age, all newborns need to be fed iron-fortified cereal and other foods rich in iron. Newborns who are formula-fed should receive iron-fortified newborn formula until 12 months of age. Mothers who breastfeed their newborns are encouraged to do so for the newborn's first 12 months of life.

    ▸ Fluoride levels in breast milk and formulas are low. A fluoride supplement should be given to newborns not receiving fluoridated water after 6 months of age.

  □ Solids are not introduced until 6 months of age. If introduced too early, food allergies can develop.

○ Breastfeeding

- Colostrum is secreted from the mother's breasts during postpartum days 1 to 3. It contains the IgA immunoglobulin that provides passive immunity to newborns.

- Breastfeeding is the optimal source of nutrition for newborns. Breastfeeding is recommended exclusively for the first 6 months of age by the American Academy of Pediatrics. Newborns should be breastfed every 2 to 3 hr. Parents should awaken the newborn to feed at least every 3 hr during the day and at least every 4 hr during the night until the newborn is feeding well and gaining weight adequately. Breastfeeding should occur 8 to 12 times within 24 hr. Then, a feed-on-demand schedule can be followed.

- Benefits of breastfeeding

  □ It reduces the risk of infection by providing IgA antibodies, lysozymes, leukocytes, macrophages, and lactoferrin that prevent infections.

  □ It promotes rapid brain growth due to large amounts of lactose.

  □ It provides protein and nitrogen for neurological cell building.

  □ Breast milk contains electrolytes and minerals.

  □ Breast milk is easy to digest, convenient, and inexpensive.

  □ It promotes maternal-infant bonding.

  □ Sucking associated with breastfeeding reduces dental and ear problems.

- Nursing interventions to promote successful breastfeeding

  □ Explain breastfeeding techniques to mothers. Have them perform hand hygiene, get comfortable, and have fluids to drink during breastfeeding.

  □ Initiate breastfeeding as soon as possible, or within the first 30 min following delivery.

  □ Explain the let-down reflex (stimulation of maternal nipple releases oxytocin that causes the letdown of milk).

  □ Reassure mothers that uterine cramps are normal during breastfeeding, resulting from oxytocin.

  □ Instruct mothers to express a few drops of colostrum or milk and spread it over the nipple to lubricate the nipple and entice the newborn.

  □ Show the mother the proper latch-on position. Have her support the breast in one hand with the thumb on top and four fingers underneath. With the newborn's mouth in front of the nipple, the newborn can be stimulated to open his mouth by tickling his lower lip with the tip of the nipple. The mother pulls the newborn to the nipple with his mouth covering part of the areola as well as the nipple.

 M ◇ View Images: Breastfeeding Techniques

  □ Explain to the mother that when her newborn is latched on correctly, his nose, cheeks, and chin will all be touching her breast.

  □ Demonstrate the four basic breastfeeding positions: football, cradle or modified cradle, across the lap, and side-lying.

- Tell mothers to feed newborns 8 to 12 times in 24 hr, usually on demand or every 2 to 3 hr. Encourage the mother to breastfeed at least 15 to 20 min/breast to ensure that newborns receive adequate fat and protein in rich hindmilk. Once the infant is feeding well and gaining weight, going to demand feeding is appropriate. Infants become more efficient at breastfeeding as they grow; consequently, the length of feedings decreases. Instructing mothers to feed for a set number of minutes is inappropriate.

- Mothers should be instructed to evaluate when the newborn has completed the feeding, including slowing of newborn suckling, a softened breast, or sleeping.

- Show the mother how to insert a finger in the side of the newborn's mouth to break the suction from the nipple prior to removing the newborn from the breast to prevent nipple trauma.

- Show mothers how to burp newborns when alternating breasts. Newborns should be burped either over the shoulder or in an upright position with the chin supported. Mothers should gently pat newborns on the back to elicit a burp.

- Tell the mother to begin the newborn's feeding with the breast she stopped feeding with in the previous feeding.

- Explain to mothers how to tell if newborns are receiving adequate feeding (gaining weight, voiding 6 to 8 diapers a day, and contentedness between feedings).

- Explain to mothers that newborns can have loose, pale, and/or yellow stools during breastfeeding, and that this is normal.

- Tell mothers how to avoid nipple confusion in newborns by not offering supplemental formula feeding or pacifier. Supplementation can be provided using a small feeding or syringe feeding, if needed.

- If nipples are sore, express breast milk and allow it to dry on the breast. The healing properties of the breast milk will decrease soreness and help avoid cracked nipples.

- Tell mothers to always place newborns on the back after feedings.

- Provide instruction for using a breast pump and storing breast milk.

- Recommend the use of a breast pump to provide milk during periods of separation.

  □ Tell mothers that breast pumps can be manual, electric, or battery-operated, and pump directly into a bottle or freezer bag.

  □ Instruct mothers that breast milk can be stored at room temperature for 4 to 6 hr. It can be refrigerated in sterile bottles for use within 8 days, or frozen in sterile containers for 3 to 6 months. Breast milk can be stored in a deep freezer for 6 to 12 months.

  □ Tell mothers that thawing the milk in the refrigerator for 24 hr is the best way to preserve the immunoglobulins present in it. It also can be thawed by holding the container under running lukewarm water or placing it in a container of lukewarm water. The bottle should be rotated often, but not shaken when thawing in this manner.

- Tell mothers that thawing by microwave is contraindicated, because it destroys some of the immune factors and lysozymes contained in the milk. Microwave thawing also leads to the development of uneven hot spots in the milk because of uneven heating, which can burn the newborn.

  □ Instruct mothers not to refreeze thawed milk.

  □ Tell mothers to discard used portions of breast milk.

  □ Recommend that mothers avoid consuming alcohol and limit caffeine.

  □ Recommend that mothers only take medications prescribed by the provider.

○ Bottle-feeding

  - Formula feeding can be a successful and adequate source of nutrition if the mother chooses not to breastfeed. The newborn should be fed every 3 to 4 hr. Parents should awaken the newborn to feed at least every 3 hr during the day and at least every 4 hr during the night until the newborn is feeding well and gaining weight adequately. Then, a feed-on-demand schedule can be followed.

  - Nursing interventions to promote successful bottle-feeding

    □ Reinforce to parents how to prepare formula, bottles, and nipples.

    □ Reinforce to parents about the different forms of formula (ready-to-feed, concentrated, and powder) and how to prepare each correctly.

    □ Instruct parents to put bottles in the dishwasher or wash by hand in hot soapy water using a good bottle and nipple brush.

    □ Reinforce to parents to wipe the lid clean on the concentrated formula can before opening it.

    □ Instruct parents to use tap water to mix concentrated or powder formula. If the water source is questionable, tap water should be boiled first.

- □ Instruct parents that prepared formula can be refrigerated for up to 48 hr.

- □ Instruct parents to check the flow of formula from the bottle to ensure it is not coming out too slow or too fast.

- □ Show parents how to cradle newborns in their arms in a semi-upright position. Newborns should not be placed in the supine position during bottle feeding because of the danger of aspiration. Newborns who bottle-feed do best when held close and at a 45° angle.

- □ Instruct parents how to place the nipple on top of the newborn's tongue, to keep the nipple filled with formula to prevent the newborn from swallowing air, and to always hold the bottle and never prop it.

 Instruct parents to burp newborns several times during a feeding, usually after each ½ to 1 oz of formula.

- □ Tell parents to place newborns in a supine position after feedings.

- □ Tell parents to discard any unused formula remaining in the bottle when newborns are finished feeding due to the possibility of bacterial contamination.

- □ Reinforce to parents how to tell if their newborn is being adequately fed (gaining weight, voiding 6 to 8 diapers per day, and satisfaction between feedings).

○ Interventions for newborns at risk for receiving inadequate nutrition

- ▪ Instruct parents who have newborns who are sleepy to:

- □ Unwrap the newborn.

- □ Change the newborn's diaper.

- □ Hold the newborn upright, and turn him from side to side.

- □ Talk to the newborn.

- □ Massage the newborn's back, and rub his hands and feet.

- □ Apply a cool cloth to the newborn's face.

- ▪ Instruct parents who have newborns who are fussy to:

- □ Swaddle them.

- □ Hold them close, move, and rock them gently.

- □ Reduce the environmental stimuli.

- □ Place them skin to skin.

- ▪ Ensure positioning and latch-on during breastfeeding is correct. Check for maternal allergy to dairy products if a breastfed newborn is spitting up, and check for an allergy or intolerance to cow's milk-based formula if a bottle-fed newborn is spitting up.

○ Elimination

- ▪ Inform parents that newborns should have 6 to 8 wet diapers a day with adequate feedings and can have 3 to 4 stools per day.

- ▪ Instruct parents to keep the newborn's diaper area clean and dry. Recommend changing the newborn's diaper frequently, cleaning the perineal area with warm water or wipes, and drying thoroughly to prevent skin breakdown. Apply barrier cream if skin becomes irritated.

○ Cord care

  ■ Instruct parents to:

    □ Keep the cord dry, and keep the top of the diaper folded underneath it.

    □ Avoid submerging newborns in water until the cord falls off around 10 to 14 days after birth. Give sponge baths until the cord falls off.

    □ Report any foul-smelling, purulent drainage or redness at the cord site to the provider.

○ Circumcision care

  ■ Circumcision is the surgical removal of the foreskin of the penis.

  ■ Circumcision should not be done immediately following birth because the newborn's level of vitamin K, which prevents hemorrhage, is at a low point. The newborn would be at risk for bleeding.

  ■ Anesthesia is required for circumcision. Types of anesthesia include a ring block, dorsal-penile nerve block, and topical anesthetic (eutectic mixture of local anesthetics). Oral sucrose, oral acetaminophen, and nonpharmacologic methods, such as swaddling and nonnutritive sucking, can be used prior to the procedure.

  ■ The presence of hypospadias (abnormal positioning of urethra on ventral undersurface of the penis) and epispadias (urethral canal terminates on dorsum of penis) are contraindications because the prepuce skin can be needed for surgical repair of the defect. Blood disorders, such as hemophilia, also are contraindications due to the increased risk for bleeding.

  ■ Yellen, Mogen, and Gomco clamp procedures

    □ The provider applies the Yellen, Mogen, or Gomco clamp to the penis, loosens the foreskin, and inserts the cone under the foreskin to provide a cutting surface for removal of the foreskin and to protect the penis.

    □ The wound is covered with sterile petroleum gauze to prevent infection and control bleeding.

  ■ Plastibell procedure

    □ The provider slides the Plastibell device between the foreskin and the glans of the penis and then ties a suture tightly around the foreskin at the coronal edge of the glans. This applies pressure, as the excess foreskin is removed from the penis.

    □ After 5 to 7 days, the Plastibell drops off, leaving a clean, well-healed excision.

    □ No petroleum is used for circumcision with the Plastibell.

> 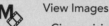 View Images
>
> › Circumcision Gomco Clamp   › Circumcision Plastibell

  ■ Preprocedure

    □ Nursing actions

      ▶ Collect data to determine any contraindications for the procedure (family history of bleeding tendencies [hemophilia and clotting disorders], acute illness, infection, hypospadias, or epispadias).

      ▶ Verify that informed consent has been given.

      ▶ Keep newborns who are bottle feeding NPO for up to 4 hr prior to the procedure or per facility policy. Breastfed newborns can eat up until the start of the procedure.

- Client education

  - Explain the procedure to the parents and assure them that an anesthetic will be administered to minimize pain.

  - Explain that the newborn will need to be restrained on a special board during the procedure.

- Intraprocedure

  - Nursing actions

    - Gather and prepare supplies.

    - Assist with procedure by:

      ▷ Placing the newborn on the restraining board and restraining the newborn's arms and legs. Do not leave the newborn unattended. Have a bulb syringe readily available.

      ▷ Assisting the provider and comforting the newborn as needed.

      ▷ Documenting in the nurse's notes circumcision type, date, and time; parent teaching reinforced; any excessive bleeding; and time newborn voids before discharge.

- Postprocedure care

  - Nursing actions

    - Remove the newborn from the restraining board.

    - Apply a diaper loosely to prevent pressure on the circumcised area.

    - Check the newborn for bleeding every 15 min for the first hour and then every hour for at least 12 hr.

    - Ensure the newborn voids.

- Client education

  - Reinforce to the parents to keep the area clean. Instruct parents to change the newborn's diaper at least every 4 hr and clean the penis with warm water with each diaper change.

  - Instruct parents following clamp procedures to apply petroleum jelly with each diaper change for at least 24 hr after the circumcision to keep the diaper from adhering to the penis.

  - Tell parents to apply the diaper loosely to prevent pressure on the circumcised area.

  - Instruct parents not to give the newborn a tub bath until the circumcision is completely healed. Until then, warm water should be trickled gently over the penis.

  - Tell the parents that a film of yellowish mucus can form over the glans by day 2, and that it is important not to wash it off.

  - Reinforce to the parents to avoid using premoistened towelettes to clean the penis because they contain alcohol.

  - Inform the parents that the newborn can be fussy or might sleep for several hours after the circumcision.

  - Inform the parents that the circumcision will heal completely within a couple of weeks.

  - Instruct the parents to notify the provider if there is any redness, discharge, swelling, strong odor, tenderness, decrease in urination, or excessive crying from the newborn.

- Complications

  - Hemorrhage

- Nursing actions
  - Monitor the newborn for bleeding.
  - Provide gentle pressure on the penis using 4 x 4 gauze. Gelfoam powder or a sponge can be applied to stop bleeding. If bleeding persists, notify the provider that a blood vessel can need to be ligated. One nurse should continue to hold pressure until the provider arrives, while another nurse prepares the circumcision tray and suture material.
  - Provide adequate discharge instructions to the parents about manifestations to observe for and how to report them to the provider.
- Clothing
  - Instruct the parents about how to properly clothe their newborn. The best clothing is soft and made of cotton. Clothes should be washed separately with mild detergent and hot water. Dress the newborn lightly for indoors and on hot days. Too many layers of clothing or blankets can make the newborn too hot. On cold days, cover the newborn's head when outdoors. A general rule is to dress the newborn as the parents would dress themselves.
- Swaddling
  - Suggest to the parents to swaddle newborns snugly in a receiving blanket to help the newborn to feel more secure.
- Safety
  - Reinforce teaching to parents regarding safety for newborns.
  - Instruct the parents to:
    - Never leave newborns unattended with pets or other small children.
    - Keep small objects (coins) out of the reach of newborns (choking hazard).
    - Never leave newborns alone on a bed, couch, or table. Newborns move enough to reach the edge and fall off.
    - Provide a firm mattress for newborns to sleep on. Never put pillows, large floppy toys, or loose plastic sheeting in a crib. The newborn can suffocate.
    - Not tie anything around the newborn's neck.
    - Monitor the safety of the newborn's crib. The space between the mattress and sides of the crib should be less than 2 fingerbreadths. The slats on the crib should be no more than 5.7 cm (2.25 in) apart.
    - Keep the newborn's crib or playpen away from window blinds and drapery cords. Newborns can become strangled in them.
    - Place the bassinet or crib near an inner wall, not next to a window, to prevent cold stress by radiation.
    - Not leave an infant carrier on a high place unattended.
    - Never leave newborns alone during bath time.
    - Have all visitors perform hand hygiene before touching newborns.
    - Keep any individual with an infection away from newborns.
    - Carefully handle newborn. Do not throw newborns up in the air or swing him by his extremities.

- Encourage parents to:

  ▸ Have smoke detectors on every floor of a home and to check them monthly to ensure that they are working. Batteries should be changed yearly. (Change batteries when daylight savings time occurs or on a child's birthday.)

  ▸ Eliminate potential fire hazards. Keep cribs and playpens away from heaters, radiators, and heat vents. Linens could catch fire if they come into contact with heat sources.

  ▸ Control the temperature and humidity of the newborn's environment by providing adequate ventilation.

  ▸ Avoid exposing the newborn to cigarette smoke in a home or elsewhere. Secondhand exposure increases the newborn's risk of developing respiratory illnesses.

- Car seat safety

  □ Instruct the parents to use an approved rear-facing car seat in the back seat, preferably in the middle (away from air bags and side impact), to transport the newborn. Infants should be in rear-facing car seats for the first 2 years of life and until they reach the maximum height and weight for the seat. In addition, a five-point harness or T-shield should be part of the convertible restraint. Do not use a used or secondhand car seat.

- Newborn wellness checkups

  □ Advise parents that their newborn will require well-newborn checkups at 2 to 6 weeks of age, and then every 2 months until 6 months of age. Newborns who are breastfed usually have a weight check around 2 days after discharge.

  □ Review the schedule for immunizations with the parents. The nurse should stress the importance of receiving these immunizations on a schedule for the newborn to be protected against diphtheria, tetanus, pertussis, hepatitis B, *Haemophilus influenzae*, polio, measles, mumps, rubella, influenza, rotavirus, pneumococcal infections, and varicella.

- Instruct the parents regarding the signs of illness and to report them immediately.

  □ A fever above 38° C (100.4° F) or a temperature below 36.6° C (97.9° F)

  □ Poor feeding or little interest in food

  □ Forceful vomiting or frequent vomiting

  □ Decreased urination

  □ Diarrhea or decreased bowel movements

  □ Labored breathing with flared nostrils or an absence of breathing for greater than 15 seconds

  □ Jaundice

  □ Cyanosis

  □ Lethargy

  □ Inconsolable crying

  □ Difficulty waking

  □ Bleeding or purulent drainage around umbilical cord or circumcision

  □ Drainage developing in eyes

APPLICATION EXERCISES

1. A nurse is preparing to administer prophylactic eye ointment into the eyes of a newborn to treat ophthalmia neonatorum. Which of the following medications should the nurse anticipate administering?

   A. Ofloxacin (Floxin)

   B. Nystatin (Mycostatin)

   C. Erythromycin (Romycin)

   D. Ceftriaxone (Rocephin)

2. A nurse is providing care for a newborn immediately after birth. Which of the following nursing actions is the highest priority?

   A. Initiating breastfeeding

   B. Performing the initial bath

   C. Administering a vitamin K injection

   D. Covering the newborn's head with a cap

3. A charge nurse is educating a newly licensed nurse regarding the administration of vitamin K (Aquamephyton) to a newborn. Which of the following is appropriate to include in the teaching?

   A. "It assists with blood clotting."

   B. "It promotes maturation of the bowel."

   C. "It is a preventative vaccine."

   D. "It provides immunity."

4. A nurse is reinforcing teaching to a mother regarding breastfeeding. Which of the following actions by the mother indicates understanding of the teaching?

   A. The mother places a few drops of water on her nipple before feeding.

   B. The mother gently removes her nipple from the infant's mouth to break the suction.

   C. When she is ready to breastfeed, the mother gently strokes the newborn's cheek with her finger.

   D. When latched on, the infant's nose, cheek, and chin are touching the breast.

5. A nurse should be aware that which of the following are contraindications for circumcising a male newborn? (Select all that apply.)

_____ A. Hypospadias

_____ B. Hydrocele

_____ C. Family history of hemophilia

_____ D. Hyperbilirubinemia

_____ E. Epispadias

6. A nurse is leading a discussion with a group of parents on bathing a newborn. What should be included in this discussion? Use the ATI Active Learning Template: Basic Concept to complete this item to include the following sections:

A. Nursing Interventions:

- Describe two interventions that relate to general skin care.

- Describe two interventions that relate to promoting infant safety.

- Describe two interventions that relate to the correct order of giving a bath.

- Describe two interventions that prevent complications in the newborn.

APPLICATION EXERCISES KEY

1. A. INCORRECT: Ofloxacin is an antibiotic, but it is not used for ophthalmia neonatorum.

    B. INCORRECT: Nystatin is used to treat *Candida albicans*, an oral yeast infection.

    C. **CORRECT:** One medication of choice for ophthalmia neonatorum is erythromycin ophthalmic ointment 0.5%. This antibiotic provides prophylaxis against *Neisseria gonorrhoeae* and *Chlamydia trachomatis*.

    D. INCORRECT: Ceftriaxone is an antibiotic, but it is not used for ophthalmia neonatorum.

    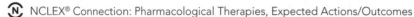 NCLEX® Connection: Pharmacological Therapies, Expected Actions/Outcomes

2. A. INCORRECT: The nurse should assist the client to initiate breastfeeding following birth, but this is not the priority action.

    B. INCORRECT: The initial bath is not given until the newborn's temperature is stable.

    C. INCORRECT: Vitamin K can be given immediately after birth, but it is not the priority action.

    D. **CORRECT:** The greatest risk to the newborn is cold stress. Therefore, the highest priority intervention is to prevent heat loss. Covering the newborn's head with a cap prevents cold stress due to excessive evaporative heat loss.

    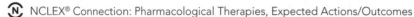 NCLEX® Connection: Health Promotion and Maintenance, Aging Process

3. A. **CORRECT:** Vitamin K is deficient in a newborn because the colon is sterile. Until bacteria are present to stimulate vitamin K production, the newborn is at risk for hemorrhagic disease.

    B. INCORRECT: Vitamin K does not assist the bowel to mature.

    C. INCORRECT: Vitamin K is a vaccine.

    D. INCORRECT: Vitamin K does not provide immunity.

    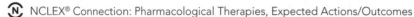 NCLEX® Connection: Health Promotion and Maintenance, Ante/Intra/Postpartum and Newborn Care

4. A. INCORRECT: The infant is enticed to suck when the mother spreads colostrum on the nipple.

    B. INCORRECT: The mother should insert a finger in the side of the newborn's mouth to break the suction before removing her nipple.

    C. INCORRECT: The mother should stroke the newborn's lips with her nipple to promote sucking.

    D. **CORRECT:** Effective latching-on includes the infant's nose, cheek, and chin touching the mother's breast.

    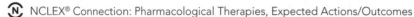 NCLEX® Connection: Health Promotion and Maintenance, Ante/Intra/Postpartum and Newborn Care

5. A. **CORRECT:** Hypospadias involves a defect in the location of the urethral opening and is a contraindication to circumcision.

    B. INCORRECT: Hydrocele, a collection of fluid in the scrotal sac, is not a contraindication to circumcision.

    C. **CORRECT:** A family history of hemophilia is a contraindication for circumcision.

    D. INCORRECT: Hyperbilirubinemia is not a contraindication for circumcision.

    E. **CORRECT:** Epispadias involves a defect in the location of the urethral opening and is a contraindication to circumcision.

    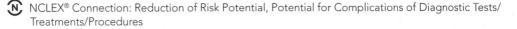 NCLEX® Connection: Reduction of Risk Potential, Potential for Complications of Diagnostic Tests/ Treatments/Procedures

6. Using ATI Active Learning Template: Basic Concept

    A. Nursing Interventions
      - Skin Care
        ○ The eyes are cleaned using a clean portion of the wash cloth.
        ○ The newborn should be washed, rinsed, and dried with no soap left on the skin.
        ○ Use a mild soap that does not contain hexachlorophene.
      - Infant Safety
        ○ Do not leave the newborn unattended during the bath.
        ○ Hot water heater should be set at 49° C (120.2° F) or lower.
        ○ The room should be warm, and the bath water should be at 36.6° to 37.2° C (97.9° to 99° F).
        ○ Bath water should be tested on the inner wrist prior to use.
      - Order of Giving the Bath
        ○ Move from the cleanest to the dirtiest areas of the newborn's body, which includes starting with the eyes, face, and head. Proceed to the chest, arms, and legs. Wash the groin area last.
        ○ The eyes are cleaned by moving from the inner to the outer canthus.
      - Preventing Complications
        ○ Bathing by immersion is not done until the umbilical cord falls off and the circumcision is healed.
        ○ To prevent spitting up and vomiting, do not bathe the newborn immediately after feeding.
        ○ After cleansing the uncircumcised newborn male, the foreskin should not be forced back.
        ○ In female newborns, wash the vulva by wiping from front to back.
        ○ Do not use lotions, oils, or powders.

    N NCLEX® Connection: Health Promotion and Maintenance, Ante/Intra/Postpartum and Newborn Care

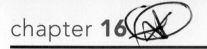

chapter 16

Overview

- Newborns can experience complications following birth. Data collection findings often are not specific, and it can be difficult to identify the cause. Complications can be discovered during routine care of newborns. Complications include prematurity, small-for-gestational-age (SGA) newborn, large-for-gestational-age (LGA)/macrosomic newborn, postterm newborn, respiratory distress syndrome, substance withdrawal, fetal alcohol syndrome, infection, cold stress, and hypoglycemia.

Risk Factors

MATERNAL RISK FACTORS	
› Diabetes mellitus	› Smoking
› Epidural anesthesia	› Preterm labor, history of preterm delivery
› Use of barbiturates or narcotics close to birth	› Abnormalities of the uterus
› Bleeding disorders	› Cervical incompetence
› Gestational hypertension	› Premature rupture of the membranes
› Multiple pregnancies	› Infections – TORCH, UTI, HIV
› Adolescent pregnancy	› Maternal substance abuse
› Lack of prenatal care	

NEONATAL RISK FACTORS	
› Prematurity, postmaturity	› Congenital or chromosomal anomalies
› LGA, SGA	› Infection
› Stress at birth, such as cold stress and asphyxia (meconium staining, cord prolapse, and nuchal cord)	› Genetic factors
	› Rh- or ABO-incompatibility

- Objective Data

  - Physical findings

    - Prematurity – A newborn born after 20 weeks of gestation and before 37 weeks of gestation is considered a preterm newborn. Preterm newborns are at risk for a variety of complications due to immature organ systems including respiratory distress syndrome (RDS), bronchopulmonary dysplasia, aspiration, intraventricular hemorrhage, retinopathy of prematurity, patent ductus arteriosus, and necrotizing enterocolitis (NEC).

      - The New Ballard score shows a physical and neuromuscular assessment of the premature infant.

      - Manifestations of increased respiratory effort or respiratory distress include nasal flaring or retractions of the chest wall during inspirations; expiratory grunting; tachypnea; cyanosis; periods of apnea longer than 10 to 15 seconds; and periodic breathing consisting of 5- to 10-second respiratory pauses, followed by 10 to 15-second compensatory rapid respirations.

      - Low birth weight with large head in comparison to total body size

- □ Minimal subcutaneous fat deposit with wrinkled features
- □ Weak reflexes including grasp, suck, swallow, gag and cough
- □ Hypotonic muscles, decreased level of activity, lethargy, and a weak cry
- SGA describes newborns whose birth weight is at or below the 10th percentile. Common complications of infants who are SGA are perinatal asphyxia, meconium aspiration, hypoglycemia, polycythemia, and instability of body temperature.
  - □ Weight below 10th percentile, normal skull, but reduced body dimensions
  - □ Wide skull sutures from inadequate bone growth
  - □ Dry, loose skin, decreased subcutaneous fat, decreased muscle mass, particularly over the cheeks and buttocks
  - □ Thin, dry, yellow, and dull umbilical cord rather than gray, glistening, and moist
  - □ Hypotonia
- LGA, or macrosomia, describes newborns whose birth weight is above the 90th percentile or more than 4,000 g (8 lb, 12 oz). LGA newborns are at risk for birth injuries (shoulder dystocia, clavicle fracture or a cesarean birth, asphyxia, hypoglycemia, polycythemia and Erb-Duchenne paralysis due to birth trauma).
  - □ Weight above 90th percentile (4,000 g)
  - □ Plump and full-faced (Cushingoid appearance) from increased subcutaneous fat
  - □ Manifestations of hypoxia including tachypnea, retractions, cyanosis, nasal flaring, and grunting
  - □ Birth trauma (fractures, intracranial hemorrhage, and CNS injury)
  - □ Sluggishness, hypotonic muscles, and hypoactivity
- Postterm newborn
  - □ Wasted appearance, thin with loose skin, having lost some of the subcutaneous fat; most of the vernix has been lost
  - □ Peeling, cracked, and dry skin; leathery from decreased protection of vernix and amniotic fluid
  - □ Long, thin body
  - □ Meconium staining of fingernails and umbilical cord
  - □ Hair and nails can be long
  - □ Macrosomia
- ○ Laboratory tests
  - Blood glucose
    - □ Confirmation of hypoglycemia – Two consecutive serum glucose levels less than 40 mg/dL in a newborn who is term
  - Culture and sensitivity of the blood, urine, and cerebrospinal fluid, positive blood cultures, usually polymicrobial (more than one pathogen) indicates the presence of infection/sepsis.
  - Serum bilirubin – direct and indirect
  - A direct Coombs test reveals the presence of antibody-coated (sensitized) Rh-positive RBCs in the newborn.

- CBC can show polycythemia (Hct greater than 65%) from in-utero hypoxia.
  - A maternal and newborn blood type is done to determine if there is a presence of ABO incapability. This occurs if the newborn has blood type A, B, or AB, and the mother is type O.
- Serum electrolytes
  - Serum calcium – hypocalcemia from long and difficult birth
- Drug screen of urine identifies suspected maternal drug use.
- Diagnostic procedures
  - ABGs
  - Chest x-ray to rule out meconium aspiration syndrome, congenital heart defects

Patient Centered Care

- Nursing Care for All Newborns
  - Monitor vital signs, I&O, and daily weight.
  - Observe skin turgor, mucous membranes, and fontanels for signs of dehydration.
  - Provide adequate nutrition.
  - Initiate early feedings.
  - Monitor the newborn's ability to suck, swallow, and digest nutrients.
  - Administer frequent, small feedings of high-calorie formula. Newborn can need gavage feedings.
  - Maintain adequate hydration.
  - Elevate the infant's head during and following feedings, and burp him to reduce vomiting and aspiration.
  - Have suction available to reduce the risk for aspiration.
  - Provide a neutral thermal environment for newborns (isolette or radiant heat warmer) to prevent cold stress.
  - Provide skin and mouth care.
  - Observe the newborn's behavior.
  - Reduce external stimuli. Touch newborns very smoothly and lightly. Keep lighting dim and noise levels low.
    - Cluster nursing care. Provide care to conserve the newborn's energy.
      - Swaddle newborns to reduce self-stimulation and protect the skin from abrasions.
      - For newborns who are addicted to cocaine, use vertical rocking and a pacifier.
  - Monitor newborns for bleeding from puncture sites and the gastrointestinal tract.
  - Administer oxygen as prescribed.
  - Monitor newborns receiving IV fluids.
  - Provide for nonnutritive sucking, such as using a pacifier while gavage feeding.
  - Protect newborns against infection by using standard precautions, performing hand hygiene and using gowns. Provide individualized equipment for newborns such as a thermometer and stethoscope.
  - Support respiratory efforts and suction the newborn as necessary to maintain an open airway.
  - Monitor the newborn's visitors for infection.

RESPIRATORY DISTRESS SYNDROME

Overview

- Respiratory distress syndrome (RDS) occurs as a result of surfactant deficiency in the lungs and is characterized by poor gas exchange and ventilatory failure.
  - ○ Objective Data
    - ■ Data collection findings
      - □ Tachypnea (respiratory rate greater than 60/min)
      - □ Nasal flaring
      - □ Expiratory grunting
      - □ Intercostal and substernal retractions
      - □ Labored breathing
      - □ Fine rales on auscultation
      - □ Cyanosis
      - □ Unresponsiveness, flaccidity, and apnea with decreased breath sounds (clinical manifestations of worsened RDS)

Patient Centered Care

- Suction the infant's mouth, trachea, and nose as needed.
- Maintain thermoregulation.
- Provide mouth and skin care.

NEONATAL SUBSTANCE WITHDRAWAL

Overview

- Substance withdrawal in the newborn occurs when the mother uses drugs that have addictive properties during pregnancy. This includes illegal drugs, alcohol, tobacco, and prescription drugs. Newborns can experience withdrawal symptoms from substances or fetal alcohol syndrome (FAS), which results from the chronic or periodic intake of alcohol during pregnancy.

Data Collection

- Objective data
  - ○ Data collection findings
    - ■ Monitor the neonate for abstinence syndrome (withdrawal) and increased wakefulness using the neonatal abstinence scoring system that assesses for and scores the following.
      - □ CNS – Increased wakefulness; sleep pattern disturbances; a high-pitched, shrill cry; incessant crying; irritability; tremors; hyperactive; increased or decreased Moro reflex; hypersensitivity to sound and external stimuli; increased deep-tendon reflexes; increased muscle tone; abrasions or excoriations on the face and knees; and seizures.

□ Metabolic, vasomotor, and respiratory findings – Nasal congestion with flaring, frequent yawning, skin mottling, respirations greater than 60/min, sweating, and hypothermia or hyperthermia.

□ Gastrointestinal – Poor feeding; poor weight gain; dehydration; regurgitation (projectile vomiting); diarrhea; and excessive, uncoordinated, constant sucking.

- Fetal Alcohol Syndrome

  □ Objective data

    ▸ Data collection findings

      ▷ Facial anomalies include eyes with epicanthal folds, strabismus, and ptosis; mouth with a poor suck, small teeth, and cleft lip or palate

      ▷ Deafness

      ▷ Abnormal palmar creases and irregular hair

      ▷ Many vital organ anomalies, such as heart defects, including atrial and ventricular septal defects, tetralogy of Fallot, and patent-ductus arteriosus

      ▷ Developmental delays and neurologic abnormalities

      ▷ Prenatal and postnatal growth retardation

      ▷ Sleep disturbances

Patient Centered Care

- Monitor the newborn's ability to feed and digest intake.
- Monitor the newborn's fluids and electrolytes such as skin turgor, mucous membranes, fontanels, and I&O.
- Observe the newborn's behavior.

NEONATAL INFECTION/SEPSIS (SEPSIS NEONATORUM)

Overview

- Infection can be contracted by newborns before, during, or after delivery. Neonatal sepsis is the presence of micro-organisms or their toxins in the blood or tissues of the infant during the first month after birth. Organisms responsible for neonatal infections include *Staphylococcus aureus*, *S. epidermidis*, *Escherichia coli*, *Haemophilus influenzae*, and *Streptococcus* ß-hemolytic, Group B.

  ○ Neonatal infection/sepsis (Sepsis Neonatorum)

  ○ Objective data

    - Data collection findings

      □ Temperature instability

      □ Suspicious drainage (eyes, umbilical stump)

      □ Poor feeding pattern, such as a weak suck or decreased intake

      □ Vomiting and diarrhea

- ☐ Poor weight gain
- ☐ Abdominal distention, large residual if feeding by gavage
- ☐ Apnea, sternal retractions, grunting, and nasal flaring
- ☐ Decreased oxygen saturation
- ☐ Color changes such as pallor, jaundice, and petechiae
- ☐ Tachycardia or bradycardia
- ☐ Tachypnea
- ☐ Low blood pressure
- ☐ Irritability and seizure activity
- ☐ Poor muscle tone and lethargic

COLD STRESS

Overview

- Cold stress (complication of ineffective thermoregulation) can lead to hypoxia, acidosis, and hypoglycemia. Newborns who have RDS are at a higher risk for hypothermia.
  - ○ Objective data
    - ■ Data collection findings
      - ☐ Drop in temperature is first sign.
      - ☐ Respiratory rate starts to increase, and then apneic spells occur.
      - ☐ Heart rate starts to increase, followed by bradycardia.
      - ☐ Skin appears mottled with acrocyanosis that can become cyanotic.
      - ☐ Physical activity is dependent on respiratory distress. Respiratory distress causes newborns to have decreased activity, whereas increased activity occurs with newborns who do not have respiratory distress.

Patient Centered Care

- Check the newborn's axillary temperature every hour until it becomes stable.
- Report an axillary temperature of less than 36.5° C (97.7° F).
- If temperature is unstable, place newborns in a radiant warmer and maintain skin temperature at approximately 36.5° C (97.7° F).
- Perform all procedures on newborns under a radiant warmer. Practice techniques to minimize heat loss (warm equipment before placing on the newborn's skin, keep bassinets away from windows).
- If cold stress does occur, warm newborns slowly over a period of 2 to 4 hr, administer oxygen, and provide for feeding to prevent hypoglycemia.

- Medications
  - Phenobarbital (Solfoton)
    - Anticonvulsant to decrease CNS irritability and control seizures for newborns who have alcohol or opioid addiction.
    - Nursing consideration – Monitor newborns for seizure activity.
  - Beractant (Survanta)
    - Lung surfactant to manage RDS and improve respiratory status
  - Betamethasone (Celestone)
    - Glucocorticoids are administered for a 24-hr period prior to delivery to promote fetal lung development and increase surfactant in an attempt to prevent RDS.
  - Ampicillin (Principen)
    - Antibiotic used for broad-spectrum bactericidal effect
    - Nursing consideration – Ensure blood cultures have been obtained prior to administration of antibiotics.
  - Gentamicin sulfate
    - Aminoglycoside antibiotic
    - Nursing Consideration – Ensure blood cultures have been obtained prior to administration of antibiotics.
  - Teamwork and collaboration
    - Request referral for home health nursing care.
    - Request referral for community support services.

HYPERBILIRUBINEMIA

Overview

- Hyperbilirubinemia is an elevation of serum bilirubin levels resulting in jaundice. Jaundice normally appears on the head (especially the sclera and mucous membranes), and then progresses down the thorax, abdomen, and extremities.
- Jaundice can be either physiologic or pathologic.
  - Physiologic jaundice is considered benign (resulting from normal newborn physiology of increased bilirubin production due to the shortened lifespan and breakdown of fetal RBCs and liver immaturity). The infant who has physiologic jaundice has no other manifestations and shows indications of jaundice after 24 hr of age.
  - Pathologic jaundice is a result of an underlying disease. Pathologic jaundice appears before 24 hr of age or is persistent after 10 days. In the term infant, bilirubin levels increase 0.5 mg/dL or more over a 4- to 8-hr period, peaks at greater than 15 mg/dL, or is associated with anemia and hepatosplenomegaly. Pathologic jaundice usually is caused by a blood group incompatibility or an infection, but can be the result of RBC disorders.

- Kernicterus (bilirubin encephalopathy) can result from untreated hyperbilirubinemia with bilirubin levels at or higher than 25 mg/dL. Bilirubin deposits in brain cells can lead to cerebral palsy, epilepsy, or mental retardation.
- Objective Data
  - Data collection findings

    - Blanching of skin on cheek or abdomen reveals yellowish tint to skin. Sclera and mucous membranes also can have yellowish tint.
    - Clinical manifestations of kernicterus
      - Very yellowish or orange skin
      - Lethargy
      - Hypotonic
      - Poor suck reflex
      - Increased sleepiness
      - If untreated, hypertonicity with backward arching of the neck and trunk
      - High-pitched cry
      - Fever

Patient-Centered Care

- Set up phototherapy if prescribed for serum bilirubin greater than 15 mg/dL prior to 48 hr of age, greater than 18 mg/dL prior to 72 hr of age, or greater than 20 mg/dL at any time.
  - Place an eye mask over the newborn's eyes after they are gently closed to protect the corneas and retinas. Ensure the nares are not covered.
  - Keep newborns undressed except for a surgical mask (make like a bikini) placed over the genitalia to prevent possible damage from heat and light waves. Be sure to remove the metal strip from the mask to prevent burning.
  - Avoid applying lotions or ointments to newborns because they absorb heat and can cause burns.
  - Remove newborns from phototherapy every 4 hr and unmask the newborn's eyes, checking for manifestations of inflammation or injury.
  - Reposition newborns every 2 hr to expose all of the body surfaces to the phototherapy lights and prevent pressure sores.
  - Check the lamp energy with a photometer per unit protocol.
  - Turn off the phototherapy lights before drawing blood for testing.
- Observe newborns for side effects of phototherapy.
  - Maculopapular skin rash of papules (small raised bumps) and macules (flat discolored areas of the skin) – usually self-limiting
  - Pressure areas
  - Dehydration (poor skin turgor, dry mucous membranes, decreased urinary output)
  - Elevated temperature

- Monitor vital signs every 4 hr.
  - Monitor bilirubin levels every 4 hr until the level returns to the expected reference range.
  - Monitor elimination, noting frequency and consistency. Frequent, loose, stools can occur due to increased gastric motility from bilirubin breakdown. Provide meticulous skin care to prevent skin breakdown in the perineal area.
  - Monitor urine output. Urine can have a brown or golden color.
  - Monitor for indications of dehydration.
    - Urine output less than 1 mL/kg/hr
    - Urine-specific gravity more than 1.015
    - Weight loss
    - Dry mucous membranes
    - Poor skin turgor
    - Depressed fontanel
  - Feed newborns frequently – Every 3 to 4 hr. This will promote bilirubin excretion in the stools.
  - Continue to breastfeed the newborn. The newborn should be breastfed at least eight times in a 24-hr period. Supplementing with formula can be prescribed. Maintain adequate fluid intake to prevent dehydration.
  - Explain hyperbilirubinemia, its causes, diagnostic tests, and treatment to parents.
  - Assist with the care of newborns who are at risk for kernicterus and receiving an exchange transfusion.

HYPOGLYCEMIA

Overview
- Hypoglycemia is a serum glucose level less than 40 mg/dL for term newborns occurring in the first 3 days of life. Untreated hypoglycemia can result in seizures, brain damage, or death.

Risk Factors
- Maternal diabetes mellitus
- Preterm infant
- LGA or SGA
- Stress at birth, such as cold stress and asphyxia
- Maternal epidural anesthesia

Data Collection

- Objective Data
  - Data collection findings
    - Poor feeding
    - Jitteriness/tremors
    - Hypothermia
    - Diaphoresis
    - Weak shrill cry
    - Lethargy
    - Flaccid muscle tone
    - Seizures/coma
    - Irregular respirations
    - Cyanosis
    - Apnea
  - Laboratory tests and diagnostic procedures
    - Plasma glucose levels less than 40 mg/dL in a newborn who is term

Patient-Centered Care

- Obtain blood per heel stick for glucose monitoring within 2 hr of life. Monitor blood glucose level per facility protocol.
- Provide frequent oral and/or gavage feedings, or continuous parenteral nutrition. Encourage early breastfeeding.
- Care After Discharge
  - Client Education
    - Reinforce proper hand hygiene and other infection control measures (the use of clean bottles and nipples for each feeding, avoiding people with acute illness).
    - Provide emotional support to families.
    - Encourage families to follow up with medical appointments.

APPLICATION EXERCISES

1. A nurse is called to the birthing room to assist with the data collection of a newborn who was delivered at 32 weeks of gestation. The newborn's birth weight is 1,100 g. Which of the following are expected findings in this newborn? (Select all that apply.)

_____ A. Lanugo

_____ B. Long nails

_____ C. Weak grasp reflex

_____ D. Translucent skin

_____ E. Plump face

2. A nurse is examining a newborn who was delivered at 41 weeks of gestation. Which of the following characteristics indicates that this newborn is postterm?

A. Excess body fat

B. Flat areola without breast buds

C. Heels movable fully to the ears

D. Leathery skin

3. A nurse is caring for an infant who has a high bilirubin level and is receiving phototherapy. Which of the following is the priority finding in this newborn?

A. Conjunctivitis

B. Bronze skin discoloration

C. Sunken fontanels

D. Maculopapular skin rash

4. A nurse is collecting data on a newborn who has a blood glucose level of 30 mg/dL. Which of the following findings requires intervention?

A. Acrocyanosis

B. Diaphoresis

C. Lusty cry

D. Flexed extremities

5. A nurse is caring for a newborn who has suspected neonatal abstinence syndrome. Which of the following findings supports this diagnosis?

    A. Decreased muscle tone

    B. Continuous high-pitched cry

    C. Sleeping for 2 hr after feeding

    D. Mild tremors when disturbed

6. A nurse educator is reviewing hyperbilirubinemia with a newly hired nurse. What should the nurse educator include in this review? Use the ATI Active Learning Template: Systems Disorder to complete this item to include the following sections:

    A. Description of Disorder: Describe the difference between physiologic and pathologic jaundice and kernicterus.

    B. Data Collection: Describe the procedure that can be used to verify the presence of jaundice.

    C. Nursing Care: Describe care of the infant receiving phototherapy.

APPLICATION EXERCISES KEY

1. A. **CORRECT:** Characteristics of a preterm newborn include the presence of abundant lanugo.

    B. INCORRECT: Long nails are findings in a newborn who is postterm.

    C. **CORRECT:** A weak grasp reflex is characteristic of a preterm newborn.

    D. **CORRECT:** Skin that is thin, smooth, shiny, and translucent is a finding in a preterm newborn.

    E. INCORRECT: The nurse would observe a plump face in a newborn who is macrosomic.

    Ⓝ NCLEX® Connection: Health Promotion and Maintenance, Data Collection Techniques

2. A. INCORRECT: A newborn who is macrosomic would have excess body fat.

    B. INCORRECT: A newborn who is preterm would have flat areolas without breast buds.

    C. INCORRECT: A newborn who is preterm would have heels that are movable fully to the ears.

    D. **CORRECT:** A newborn who is postterm due to placental insufficiency would have leathery, cracked, and wrinkled skin.

    Ⓝ NCLEX® Connection: Health Promotion and Maintenance, Data Collection Techniques

3. A. INCORRECT: Conjunctivitis is an important finding, but it is not the priority.

    B. INCORRECT: Bronze skin discoloration is an important finding, but it is not the priority.

    C. **CORRECT:** Using the safety and risk-reduction framework, sunken fontanels is the priority finding. Infants receiving phototherapy are at risk for dehydration from loose stools due to increased bilirubin excretion.

    D. INCORRECT: Maculopapular skin rash is an important finding, but it is not the priority.

    Ⓝ NCLEX® Connection: Physiological Adaptations, Fluid and Electrolyte Imbalances

4. A. INCORRECT: Acrocyanosis is an expected finding in the newborn.

    B. **CORRECT:** Diaphoresis is a data collection finding associated with hypoglycemia.

    C. INCORRECT: A lusty cry is an expected finding in the newborn.

    D. INCORRECT: Flexed extremities are a normal finding seen in the newborn.

    Ⓝ NCLEX® Connection: Physiological Adaptations, Alterations in Body Systems

5. A. INCORRECT: A newborn who has neonatal abstinence syndrome can have increased muscle tone.

   B. **CORRECT:** A continuous high-pitched cry is often an indication of CNS disturbances in a newborn who has neonatal abstinence syndrome.

   C. INCORRECT: A newborn who has neonatal abstinence syndrome can have sleep pattern disturbances and would have difficulty sleeping for 2 hr after feeding.

   D. INCORRECT: A newborn who has neonatal abstinence syndrome often has moderate to severe tremors when undisturbed. Many normal newborns have mild tremors when disturbed.

   Ⓝ NCLEX® Connection: Physiological Adaptations, Alterations in Body Systems

6. *Using the ATI Active Learning Template: Systems Disorder*

   A. Description of Disorder
   - Physiologic jaundice results from the breakdown of fetal RBCs and lack of liver maturity and appears after 24 hr of age.
   - Pathologic jaundice is caused by a blood incompatibility, infection, or a disorder of RBCs, and appears before 24 hr of age.
   - Kernicterus is a neurological syndrome caused by bilirubin deposits in brain cells when bilirubin levels are very high. It can result in long-term neurological problems.

   B. Data Collection
   - Procedure to verify presence of jaundice
     ○ Press the newborn's skin on the cheek or abdomen lightly with one finger.
     ○ Then release pressure, and observe for a yellowish tint to the skin as the skin is blanched.

   C. Nursing Care
   - Care of the infant receiving phototherapy
     ○ Maintain an eye mask over the newborn's eyes.
     ○ Keep the newborn undressed. Place a mask (like a bikini) over the genitalia of a male newborn.
     ○ Remove the newborn from phototherapy every 4 hr, and unmask the eyes.
     ○ Reposition the newborn every 2 hr to expose all body surfaces to the phototherapy lights and prevent pressure sores.
     ○ Check the lamp energy with a photometer following facility protocol.
     ○ Turn off the phototherapy lights before drawing blood for testing.

   Ⓝ NCLEX® Connection: Physiological Adaptations, Alterations in Body Systems

chapter 17

Overview

- Bonding and integration of an infant into the family structure should start during pregnancy, continue into the fourth stage of labor, and throughout hospitalization.

- Assessment of bonding and integration of an infant into the family structure requires that a nurse understand the normal postpartum psychological changes the client undergoes in the attainment of the maternal role and the recognition of deviations. Baby-friendly care can be promoted by delaying nursing procedures during the first hour after birth and through the first attempt of the client to breastfeed to allow for immediate parent-infant contact.

  - A client's emotional and physical condition (unwanted pregnancy, adolescent pregnancy, history of depression, difficult pregnancy and delivery) and the infant's physical condition (prematurity, congenital anomalies) after birth can affect the family's bonding process.

  - Culture, age, and socioeconomic level can influence the bonding process.

- Bonding can be delayed secondary to maternal or neonatal factors.

Psychosocial and Maternal Adaptation

- Psychosocial adaptation and maternal adjustment begin during pregnancy as the client goes through commitment, attachment, and preparation for the birth of the newborn. During the first 2 to 6 weeks after birth, the client goes through a period of acquaintance with her newborn, as well as physical restoration. During this time, she also focuses on competently caring for her newborn. Finally, the act of achieving maternal identity is accomplished around 4 months following birth. It is important to note that these stages can overlap, and are variable based on maternal, infant, and environmental factors.

  - Phases of maternal role attainment

    - Dependent: taking-in phase

      - First 24 to 48 hr
      - Focus is on meeting personal needs
      - Rely on others for assistance
      - Excited, talkative; need to review birth experience with others

    - Dependent-independent: taking-hold phase

      - Begins on day 2 or 3; up to several weeks
      - Focus on baby care and improving caregiving competency
      - Want to take charge but need acceptance from others
      - Want to learn and practice

    - Interdependent: letting-go phase

      - Focus on family as a unit
      - Resumption of role (intimate partner, individual)

- Nursing examinations include noting the client's condition after birth, observing the maternal adaptation process, observing maternal emotional readiness to care for the infant, and observing how comfortable the client appears in providing infant care.
  - Observe for behaviors that facilitate and indicate mother-infant bonding.
    - Considers the infant a family member.
    - Holds the infant face-to-face (en face), maintaining eye contact.
    - Assigns meaning to the infant's behavior and views positively.
    - Identifies the infant's unique characteristics and relates them to those of other family members.
    - Names the infant, indicating that bonding is occurring.
    - Touches the infant and maintains close physical proximity and contact.
    - Provides physical care for the infant such as feeding and diapering.
    - Responds to the infant's cries.
    - Smiles at, talks to, and sings to the infant.
  - Monitor for behaviors that impair and indicate a lack of mother-infant bonding.
    - Apathy when the infant cries.
    - Disgust when the infant voids, stools, or spits up.
    - Expresses disappointment in the infant.
    - Turns away from the infant.
    - Does not seek close physical proximity to the infant.
    - Does not talk about the infant's unique features.
    - Handles the infant roughly.
    - Ignores the infant entirely.
  - Monitor for signs of mood swings, conflict about maternal role, and/or personal insecurity.
    - Feelings of being "down."
    - Feelings of inadequacy.
    - Feelings of anxiety related to ineffective breastfeeding.
    - Emotional lability with frequent crying.
    - Flat affect and being withdrawn.
    - Feeling unable to care for the infant.
- Nursing interventions to assist with maternal-infant bonding.
  - Facilitate the bonding process by placing the infant skin-to-skin in the en face position with the client immediately after birth.
  - Promote rooming-in as a quiet and private environment that enhances the family bonding process.
  - Promote early initiation of breastfeeding, and encourage the client to recognize infant readiness cues. Offer assistance as needed.
  - Instructing the client about infant care facilitates bonding as the client's confidence improves.
  - Encourage the parents to bond with their infant through cuddling, bathing, feeding, diapering, and inspection.
  - Provide frequent praise, support, and reassurance to the client as she moves toward independence in caring for her infant and adjusting to her maternal role.
  - Encourage parents to express their feelings, fears, and anxieties about caring for their infant.

Paternal Adaptation

- Paternal adaptation takes place as the father develops a parent-infant bond.
  - The father has skin-to-skin contact, holds, and maintains eye-to-eye contact with the infant.
  - The father observes the infant for features similar to his own to validate his claim of the infant.
  - The father talks, sings, and reads to the infant.
- Paternal transition to fatherhood consists of a predictable three-stage process during the first few weeks of transition.
  - Expectations – The father has preconceived ideas about what it will be like to be a father.
  - Reality – The father discovers that his expectations might not be met. Commonly expressed emotions include feeling sad, frustrated, and jealous. He embraces the need to be actively involved in parenting.
  - Transition to mastery – The father decides to become actively involved in the care of the infant.
- The development of the father-infant bond consists of three stages.
  - Making a commitment – The father takes the responsibility of parenting.
  - Becoming connected – The father experiences feelings of attachment to the infant.
  - Making room for the infant – The father modifies his life to include the care of the infant.
- Monitoring paternal adaptation includes observing for the characteristics of father-infant bonding.
- Nursing interventions to assist in the father-infant bonding process.
  - Provide education about infant care when the father is present, and encourage the father to take a hands-on approach.
  - Assist the father in his transition to fatherhood by providing guidance and involving him as a full partner rather than just a helper.
  - Encourage couples to verbalize their concerns and expectations related to infant care.

Sibling Adaptation

- The addition of an infant into the family unit affects everyone in the family, including siblings who can experience a temporary separation from the mother. Siblings become aware of changes in the parents' behavior because the infant requires much more of the parents' time.
- Nursing observation of sibling adaptation to the infant
  - Monitor for positive responses from the sibling.
    - Interest and concern for the infant
    - Increased independence
  - Monitor for adverse responses from the sibling.
    - Signs of sibling rivalry and jealousy
    - Regression in toileting and sleep habits
    - Aggression toward the infant
    - Increased attention-seeking behaviors and whining

- Nursing interventions to facilitate sibling acceptance of the infant
  - Take the sibling on a tour of the obstetric unit.
  - Encourage the parents to:
    - Let the sibling be one of the first to see the infant.
    - Provide a gift from the infant to give the sibling.
    - Arrange for one parent to spend time with the sibling while the other parent is caring for the infant.
    - Allow older siblings to help in providing care for the infant.
    - Provide preschoolers with a doll to care for.

Complications and Nursing Implications

- Impaired parenting can include emotional detachment and inability to care for the infant, thus placing the infant at risk for neglect and failure to thrive. Failure to bond with the infant increases the risk of physical and/or emotional abuse.
- Nursing interventions for impaired parenting
  - Emphasize verbal and nonverbal communication skills between the client, caregivers, and infant.
  - Provide continued observation of the client's parenting abilities, as well as any other caregivers for the infant.
  - Encourage the continued support of grandparents and other family members.
  - Provide home visits by a nurse and group sessions for discussion regarding infant care and parenting problems.
  - Give the client/caregivers information about social networks that provide a support system where they can seek assistance.
  - Involve outreach programs concerned with self-care, parent-child interactions, child injuries, and failure to thrive.
  - Notify programs that provide prompt and effective community interventions to prevent more serious problems from occurring.

APPLICATION EXERCISES

1. A nurse concludes that the father of an infant is not showing positive signs of parent-infant bonding and appears to be very anxious and nervous when the infant's mother asks him to bring her the infant. Which of the following is a nursing intervention to promote father-infant bonding?

    A. Hand the father the infant, and suggest that he change the diaper.

    B. Ask the father why he is so anxious and nervous.

    C. Tell the father that he will grow accustomed to the infant.

    D. Provide education about infant care when the father is present.

2. A client in the early postpartum period is very excited and talkative. She is repeatedly telling the nurse every detail of her labor and birth. Because the client will not stop talking, the nurse is having difficulty completing the postpartum examination. Which of the following interventions should the nurse perform?

    A. Come back later when the client is more cooperative.

    B. Give the client time to express her feelings.

    C. Tell the client that she needs to be quiet so the postpartum examination can be completed.

    D. Redirect the client's focus so that she will become quiet.

3. A nurse is caring for a client who is 1 day postpartum. The nurse is observing for maternal adaptation and mother-infant bonding. Which of the following behaviors by the client indicate a need for the nurse to intervene? (Select all that apply.)

    _____ A. Demonstrates apathy when the infant cries

    _____ B. Touches the infant and maintains close physical proximity

    _____ C. Views the infant's behavior as uncooperative during diaper changing

    _____ D. Identifies and relates infant's characteristics to those of family members

    _____ E. Interprets the infant's behavior as meaningful and a way of expressing needs

4. A nurse is accompanying a home-health nurse who is conducting a visit to the home of a client who has a 2-month-old infant and a 4-year-old son. The client expresses frustration about the behavior of the 4-year-old who was previously toilet trained and is now frequently wetting himself. The nurse should provide education and explains to the client that

    A. her son was probably not ready for toilet training and should wear training pants.

    B. her son is showing an adverse sibling response.

    C. this indicates the child requires counseling.

    D. this can be resolved by sending the child to preschool.

5. A nurse in the delivery room is planning to promote maternal-infant bonding for a client who just delivered. Which of the following is the priority action by the nurse?

    A. Encourage the parents to touch and explore the neonate's features.

    B. Limit noise and interruption in the delivery room.

    C. Place the neonate at the client's breast.

    D. Place the neonate skin-to-skin on the client's chest.

6. A charge nurse is leading a parenting class on paternal adaptation for expectant women and their partners. Which concepts on paternal adaptation should the nurse include in the presentation? Use ATI Active Learning Template: Basic Concept to complete this item to include the following:

    A. Related Content: Describe three ways the father develops a parent-infant bond.

    B. Underlying Principles:
- Describe three stages of paternal transition to parenthood.
- Describe three stages of the development of the father-infant bond.

    C. Nursing Interventions: Describe three actions to assist in the father-infant bonding process.

APPLICATION EXERCISES KEY

1. A. INCORRECT: It is not helpful to push the father into infant care activities without first providing education.

    B. INCORRECT: This is a nontherapeutic statement and presumes the nurse knows what the father is feeling.

    C. INCORRECT: This is a nontherapeutic statement and offers the nurse's opinion.

    D. **CORRECT:** Nursing interventions to promote paternal bonding include providing education about infant care and encouraging the father to take a hands-on approach.

    Ⓝ NCLEX® Connection: Health Promotion and Maintenance, Developmental Stages and Transitions

2. A. INCORRECT: The nurse should not delay completing the examination, but continue her activities while encouraging the client to talk.

    B. **CORRECT:** The nurse should recognize that the client in is the taking-in phase, which begins immediately following birth and lasts a few hours to a couple of days.

    C. INCORRECT: It is not necessary for the client to stop talking while the nurse completes the needed examination.

    D. INCORRECT: The client is in the taking-in phase, which includes talking about the birth experience. The client should be encouraged to talk about the birth experience.

    Ⓝ NCLEX® Connection: Health Promotion and Maintenance, Ante/Intra/Postpartum and Newborn Care

3. A. **CORRECT:** This behavior demonstrates a lack of interest in the infant and impaired maternal-infant bonding.

    B. INCORRECT: Touching the infant and maintaining close proximity are signs of effective maternal-infant bonding.

    C. **CORRECT:** A client's view of her infant as being uncooperative during diaper changing is a sign of impaired maternal-infant bonding.

    D. INCORRECT: Endowing the infant with family characteristics indicates effective maternal-infant bonding.

    E. INCORRECT: Recognizing the infant's behavior as meaningful and a way to express needs is an indication of effective maternal-infant bonding.

    Ⓝ NCLEX® Connection: Health Promotion and Maintenance, Developmental Stages and Transitions

4. A. INCORRECT: This is not an appropriate intervention by the nurse because it overlooks the child's emotional response to a new family member.

   B. **CORRECT:** Adverse responses by a sibling to a new infant can include regression in toileting habits.

   C. INCORRECT: Recommending that the child receive counseling is not an appropriate nursing intervention for an adverse sibling response.

   D. INCORRECT: Recommending that the child be sent to preschool is not an appropriate nursing intervention for an adverse sibling response.

   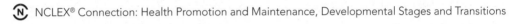 NCLEX® Connection: Health Promotion and Maintenance, Developmental Stages and Transitions

5. A. INCORRECT: Encouraging the parents to touch and explore the neonate's features is important to promote maternal-infant bonding. However, this is not the priority nursing intervention.

   B. INCORRECT: Limiting noise and interruptions in the delivery room is important to promote maternal-infant bonding. However, this is not the priority nursing intervention.

   C. INCORRECT: Placing the neonate at the client's breast is important, but this is not the priority nursing intervention.

   D. **CORRECT:** Placing the neonate in the en face position on the client's chest immediately after birth is the priority nursing intervention to promote maternal-infant bonding.

   NCLEX® Connection: Health Promotion and Maintenance, Developmental Stages and Transitions

6. *Using the ATI Active Learning Template: Basic Concept*

   A. Related Content

   - Development of parent-infant bond

      ○ Touching, holding, skin-to-skin contact, and maintaining eye-to-eye contact

      ○ Recognizing personal features in the infant, and validating his claim to the infant

      ○ Talking, reading, singing, and verbally interacting with the infant

   B. Underlying Principles

   - Stages of paternal transition to parenthood

      ○ Expectations – having preconceived ideas about fatherhood

      ○ Reality – recognizing expectations might not be met, facing these feelings, and then embracing the need to become actively involved in parenting

      ○ Transition to mastery – taking an active role in parenting

   - Development of the father-infant bond

      ○ Making a commitment and assuming responsibility for parenting

      ○ Becoming connected and having feelings of attachment to the infant

      ○ Modifying lifestyle to make room to care for the infant

   C. Nursing Interventions

   - Provide education about infant care when father is present.

   - Encourage the father to take a hands-on role in care when present.

   - Provide guidance.

   - Involve the father as a full partner, not a helper, in the parenting process.

   - Encourage the couple to verbalize their concerns and expectations about infant care.

   Ⓝ NCLEX® Connection: Health Promotion and Maintenance, Developmental Stages and Transitions

REFERENCES

Dudek, S. G. (2010). *Nutrition essentials for nursing practice* (6th ed.). Philadelphia: Lippincott Williams & Wilkins.

Grodner, M., Roth, S. L., & Walkingshaw, B. C. (2012). *Nutritional foundations and clinical applications: A nursing approach* (5th ed.). St. Louis, MO: Mosby.

Hockenberry, M. J., & Winkelstein M. L. (2013). *Wong's essentials of pediatric nursing* (9th ed.). St. Louis, MO: Mosby.

Lehne, R. A. (2013). *Pharmacology for nursing care* (8th ed.). St. Louis: Saunders.

Lowdermilk, D. L., Perry, S. E., Cahsion, M. C., & Aldean, K. R. (2012). *Maternity & women's health care* (10th ed.). St. Louis, MO: Mosby.

Perry, S. E., Hockenberry, M. J., Lowdermilk, D. L., & Wilson, D. (2010). *Maternal Child Nursing Care* (4th ed.). St. Louis, MO: Mosby Elsevier.

Pillitteri, A. (2010). *Maternal and child health nursing: Care of the childbearing and childrearing family* (6th ed.). Philadelphia: Lippincott Williams & Wilkins.

Wilson, B. A., Shannon, M. T., & Shields, K. M. (2013). *Pearson nurse's drug guide 2013*. Upper Saddle River, NJ: Prentice Hall.

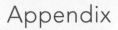

Appendix

CONTENT _____ REVIEW MODULE CHAPTER _____

TOPIC DESCRIPTOR_____

Related Content
(e.g. delegation, levels of prevention, advance directives)

Underlying Principles

Nursing Interventions
› Who?
› When?
› Why?
› How?

Appendix

CONTENT _____ REVIEW MODULE CHAPTER _____

TOPIC DESCRIPTOR _____

DESCRIPTION OF PROCEDURE:

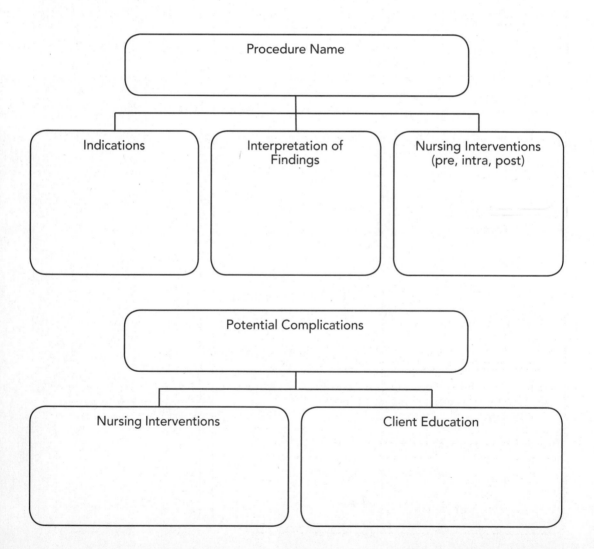

Procedure Name

Indications

Interpretation of Findings

Nursing Interventions (pre, intra, post)

Potential Complications

Nursing Interventions

Client Education

Appendix

CONTENT _____ REVIEW MODULE CHAPTER _____

TOPIC DESCRIPTOR_____

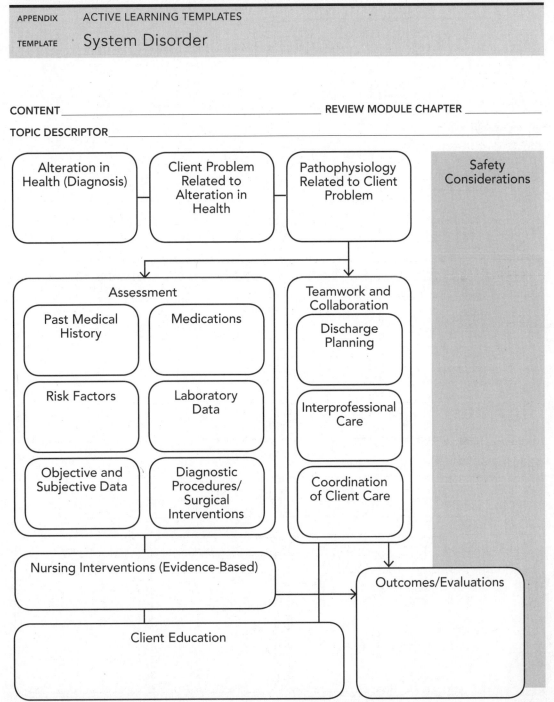

Appendix

CONTENT _____ REVIEW MODULE CHAPTER _____

TOPIC DESCRIPTOR _____

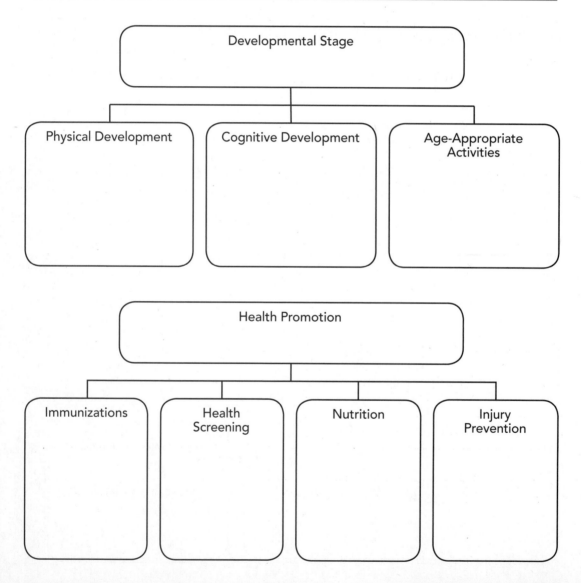

APPENDIX	ACTIVE LEARNING TEMPLATES
TEMPLATE	Medication

CONTENT _____ REVIEW MODULE CHAPTER _____

TOPIC DESCRIPTOR_____

MEDICATION _____

EXPECTED PHARMALOGICAL ACTION:

Therapeutic Uses

Adverse Effects

Nursing Interventions

Contraindications

Medication/Food Interactions

Client Education

Medication Administration

Evaluation of Medication Effectiveness

Appendix

CONTENT _____ REVIEW MODULE CHAPTER _____

TOPIC DESCRIPTOR_____

DESCRIPTION OF SKILL:

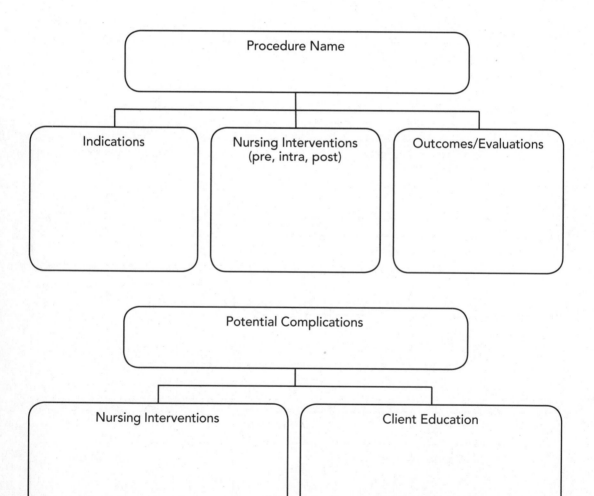

Procedure Name

Indications

Nursing Interventions (pre, intra, post)

Outcomes/Evaluations

Potential Complications

Nursing Interventions

Client Education

Appendix

APPENDIX ACTIVE LEARNING TEMPLATES

TEMPLATE Therapeutic Procedure

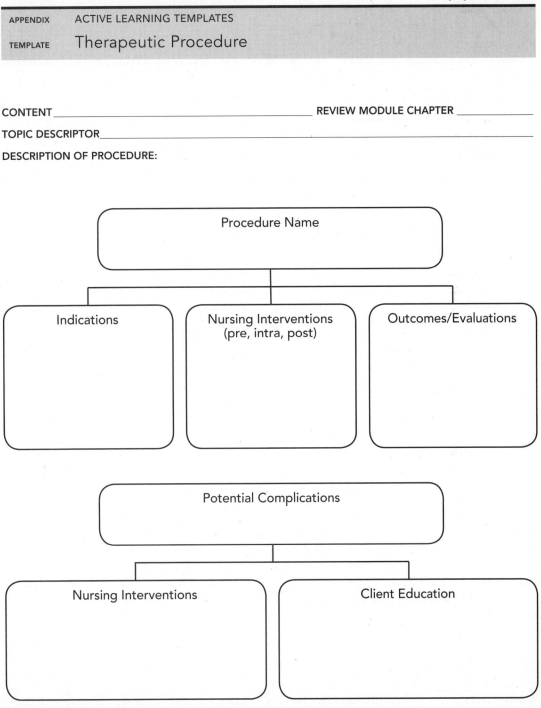

CONTENT _____ REVIEW MODULE CHAPTER _____

TOPIC DESCRIPTOR_____

DESCRIPTION OF PROCEDURE:

Procedure Name

Indications

Nursing Interventions
(pre, intra, post)

Outcomes/Evaluations

Potential Complications

Nursing Interventions

Client Education

                                    parental
① Custodio ∧ — control

② Mamabear